Who Will Be My Mother's Keeper

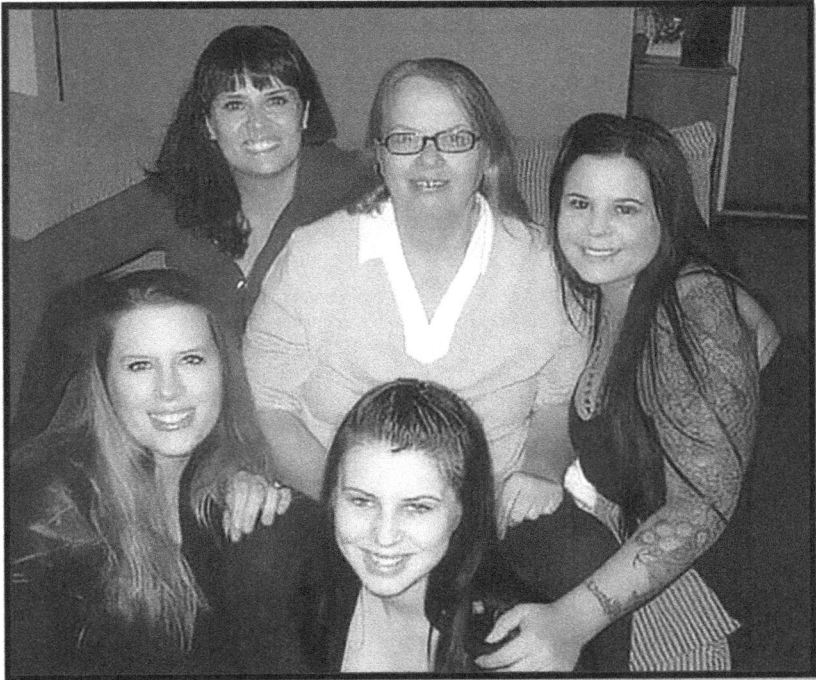

A Story of Learning & Self-Discovery

Sock Monkey Press

In the Words of
Katie Stakolich & Dr. Alfred Aidoo

As told to
Pete Hedrick & Greg Peters

Dedicated to…

The Keepers of All God's Sheep

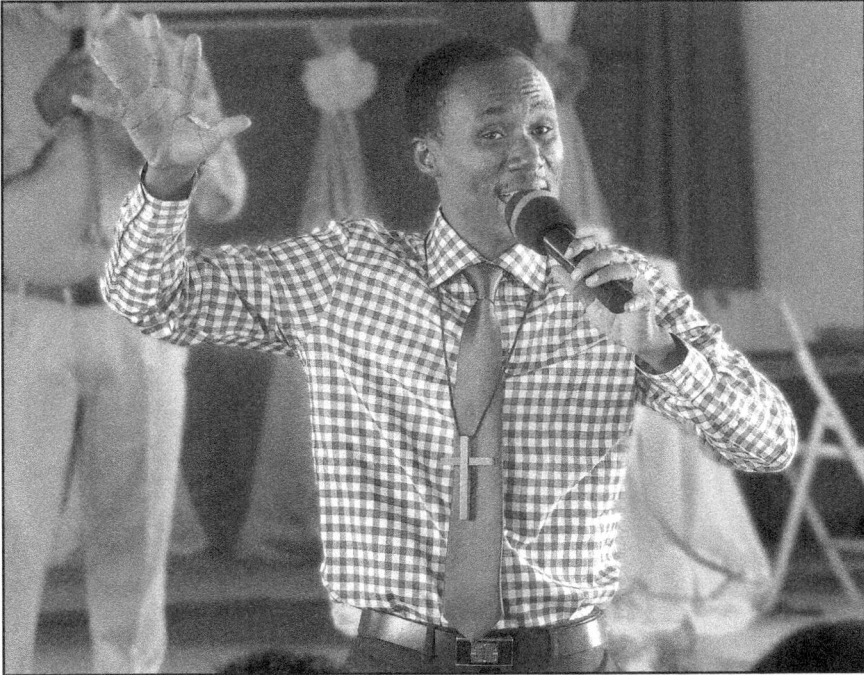

"*For what good then is a shepherd if
when his flock is lost, he cannot be found. And so, too
what good then am I as a doctor if when people are sick,
I am nowhere around?*

*Just as a good shepherd must always care enough about his
flock to carry with him the smell of his sheep. So then, I as a
shepherd of men, must always carry with me the
smell of my sheep.*"

Dr. Alfred Aidoo

Table of Contents

PREFACE:
From Different Worlds

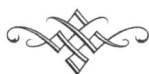

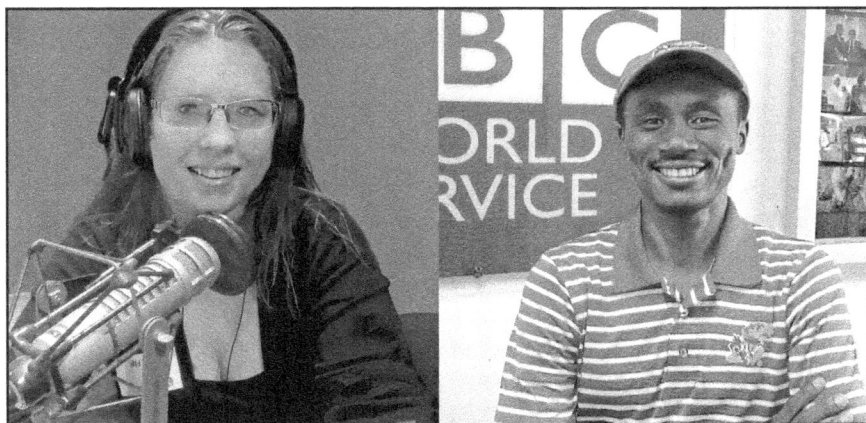

This is the curious story about how a mentally ill grandmother in her 60s from California, wound up living in Africa with the 20-something fiancé she met on the internet and how her death in a mysterious car crash would lead two total strangers into a desperate attempt to save her life all while forming a special bond that goes beyond friendship and spans two continents.

In this book, Katie Stakolich and Dr. Alfred Aidoo describe in their own words how upon finding Katie's runaway mother clinging to life in a Ghanaian hospital it would set off a tsunami of emotions so strong that they continue to color the lives of her friends and family on two continents to this day.

Until Sandra Lee Pope died from injuries suffered in car crash in

2016, there was no reason for Katie and Alfred to know each other existed. Katie was busy holding down a fulltime job at a supermarket in California, while she and her husband were busy raising two boys. Alfred, too, was leading a hectic life. As if his job as an emergency room doctor weren't enough to keep him hopping from morning until night, he also spent time minding a flock of parishioners as a minister in his church, while he and his wife were raising two young daughters of their own.

Many of the details regarding the crash that claimed the life of Katie's mother remain murky at best. Here is what we do know for sure. Katie's mother had spent months purposely trying to avoid any communication with her family. First moving to Germany and then Ghana. She had been in a car with her fiancé when it was involved in a wreck. While Sandra wound up in the emergency room with critical injuries, her fiancé suffered only minor injuries. We also know that this in turn led to Alfred becoming Sandra's emergency room doctor. And that resulted in him reaching out to find her family in the United States, and that's what brought Katie and Alfred together.

Haunted by insecurities that fueled her own manic behavior, Sandra never seemed satisfied with her life, and as a result her family bore the brunt of her rejection and abandonment. She was constantly seeking ways to escape and distance herself from a caring family, who in actuality wanted little more than for her just to be their mother.

Through his care for Sandra, Alfred was able to glean a lot about the toll her mental illness had exacted on her family. This knowledge helped him paint a clearer image of the inner workings of their family dynamics. In just a short time, he went from simply being Sandra's physician, to being her personal patient advocate, and then a trusted family confidante. In the end, he rose to become the keeper of a discordant flock of souls in a family so bent on fulfilling their own selfish desires that they weren't able to care for those closest to them in their greatest hour of need.

This is also a complex story about how the pressures of growing up with a mentally ill parent can put so much stress and strain on a family that their emotions can boil over making it a struggle simply to give the afflicted person their unconditional love. For Katie's family, the years of uncertainty and duress have meant years of packing and unpacking a lifetime of emotional baggage, which manifested themselves in physical, mental and emotional abuse, before finally giving way to renewal, forgiveness and redemption.

Katie and Alfred bravely confront their own human frailties and doubts about what it means to be human. Their voices come together to remind us how by merely taking responsibility for the well-being of just one other person you can start a ripple of compassion that that builds into a wave of caring as it washes to a distant shore.

1

The Good Samaritan

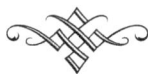

Tears flowed down my cheeks as I sat alone on my living room floor weeping while my mother lay dying in a strange hospital in an unfamiliar country halfway around the world. "I am so sorry," I mumbled over and over to myself as visions of my Mother dying all alone ran on a continuous loop in my head. "I'm so sorry this has happened to you."

This fateful chapter of my mother's chaotic jumble of a life started just weeks earlier when she was seriously injured in a mysterious car crash in Ghana – a West African country that quite frankly I had never even heard of until I caught wind of the accident. When Mom still wasn't responding to medical treatment about a week or so after the crash, her primary care doctor at Komfo Anokye Teaching Hospital called me at my home in California. "Your mom still hasn't woken up," he said. "We need to create an atmosphere that will make her feel like she is safe. Hearing your voice would be helpful."

Given my tumultuous history with my mentally ill mother throughout our lives, I knew talking to her was going to be incredibly difficult for me. But even though she had spent the last two years secretly doing everything in her power to distance herself from me and our entire family, my heart told me helping my mother was the right thing to do. However angry or upset or disappointed I had been with her over the years, I needed to set those feelings aside and do everything possible to find out if Mom was still alive. So, I braced myself for what would come next.

"What do you need me to do?" I said.

"I want you to speak with her," said Dr. Alfred Aidoo, his calm voice assuring me that I could find the strength inside me to do this. "I'll put you on speaker phone so you can talk to her. Hopefully, she will respond enough for us to see something."

Words can't begin to express the flood of emotions that ran through me as I steeled myself for what might be our last conversation, ever. I hadn't spoken to Mom in a long time, and now perhaps the most important conversation of our lives would be happening over a cellphone. Alfred sensed how emotionally challenging this moment was for me. He knew I was torn between the unconditional love a child feels for her parent, and the horrific stories I had shared with him about the friction between us that started in my childhood and continued even after I had a family of my own.

"She may not even recognize my voice," I protested.

"All the more reason for you to make the attempt," Alfred said. "You will tell her who you are, and if she recognizes you, we will know that we should continue trying to bring her out of her coma."

"OK, let's try it," I hesitantly agreed. What else could I do? This was still my mother.

"Be strong," Alfred encouraged and then put me on speakerphone with Mom and the other doctors in the room.

"Mom, this is Katie, your daughter," my voice quivered as I began to cry. "You've been in a car accident in Ghana. You are in the hospital. Alfred Aidoo is your doctor. He is there with you now. He is going to help us, but I need you to open your eyes. Just try to open them … please. Dr. Aidoo needs to see if you are still there. Can you open your eyes …Mom?

"Please? Mom, just open your eyes." I kept asking her this same thing over and over again for what felt like an eternity. "I'm sorry that I couldn't understand what you were going through. Please forgive me. I forgive you for everything that I have been holding against you all these years. I'm here for you, and I will be here every day. I will not leave you. I promise. I love you, Mom."

"Katie, your mom moved her arm a little, and her eyes are fluttering," Alfred said, hope rising in his voice.

"Did she open her eyes?" I asked.

"No, but I can tell she tried," Alfred replied, "And that is enough. I know she heard you. You did amazing! Now that we know she is still in there, we can figure out what to try next. Thank you, Katie."

"Thank you, Alfred." I said, while I continued sitting alone on the living room floor awash in my thoughts and emotionally drained. I let myself believe there that was still hope that Mom was still alive. "I am so sorry ... I'm so sorry this has happened to you."

2

Mothers And Daughters

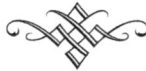

Given the unique dynamics between my mother and me throughout our lives, I see the world a little differently than most when it comes to moms and daughters. It comforts me in some strange way knowing that most girls and their mothers experience some level of friction in their relationships, which, in turn, makes me feel like maybe I'm more normal than I give myself credit for.

What teenage girl hasn't hated her mother at some point in her life? The difference for me compared to other girls is that at age 16 I actually up and left my Mom, fully convinced the split was for the for the best. I then moved in with my Dad and for much of the next three years Mom and I never saw or spoke to one another. Our relationship became so strained at that point that if someone had looked into a crystal ball back then and told me that more than two decades later, I would be fighting for her life while she was dying in Africa, I wouldn't have believed it for a second.

Recently, a girl caught me staring at her while I was working. She held my gaze for a long second before I quickly turned away and continued stocking shelves at the supermarket where I have been employed since high school. Don't worry, I'm not a danger to anyone. At the end of the day, I'm just a somewhat frazzled mom of two pre-teen boys who is trying to keep it all together. The difference is that my perspective on life is colored by a toxic history between me and my emotionally unstable, often-absent mom, especially mother-daughter relationships.

Generally speaking, however, most teenage-girl dramas don't bother me. When groups of adolescent girls come into the store, giggling with their friends and buying junk food for their slumber parties, I don't blink an eye. I see older teenage girls with their good-looking boyfriends hanging out, and it doesn't faze me in the least. The ones that really get to me are the teenage girls who come in with their moms, smiling as if they are silently sharing an inside joke with their best friends. That's when jealousy twists me into a knot of emotions. Thanks, mom.

No matter how much I would love to feel the same way about my mom as the girls who can share their secrets with just a glance, I don't. Or maybe I can't. It sounds petty, but for my sanity I'm relieved this kind of close relationship between mothers and daughters is not the norm. The teenage girls who act like buddies with their moms are the exceptions and not the rule.

It's taken me years to get to this point of grace in my life, but I know that I *truly* loved my mother. Yes, the anger, resentment and hatred still flare up from time to time. Even long after her death, I am continuing to learn how to deal with those emotions. In my heart, I know God has a plan for all of us, and my mother and her mental illness are part of His plan for me.

3

(Alfred)
I Am Alfred Jacob Aidoo

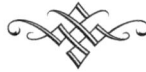

Dad loved all of life, and he did whatever he could to help others. Much of who I am today — the love I have for people and my reluctance to turn away from those who need my help — comes from my father. "Nothing is more important than caring for your fellow man and going the extra mile to tend to the needs of others," he taught my brother and me.

My father, Robert A. Aidoo, and my mother, Margaret Danso Quayson, divorced around the time when I was born. My brother, Robert, and I lived with my mother for the first couple years, but when she remarried our father grew concerned that we were not getting a good enough education, so he decided to become our primary caregiver. I cried when we left Mom's house like any young child might. Looking back now as an adult, I can better understand what my Dad did and why, and I love him for it. Don't get me wrong, I genuinely love my mother and we remain close, but most of who I am today as a person, I owe to my father.

While I am not an old man, I have always felt mature well beyond my years. Even at an early age, I spent a lot of time thinking about the struggles so many people had to endure just to survive. My father was far from immune from my concerns. When I was quite young, I began sharing the anguish I imagined he felt dealing with the challenges life set before him as a single parent with two young sons.

His composure in the face of adversity, and his grace under pressure resonated within me. Even though I did not realize it at the time, simply watching the way Dad dealt with all the challenges we faced throughout my childhood was laying the groundwork for who I am today. In many important ways, Dad's treatment of others taught me the greatest moral and ethical lessons a developing young mind like mine could have had. I have no doubt these experiences forged were critical in forming the foundation of who I am today.

School was one of the main places where I could noticeably feel the gap between the reality of *our* family's existence and the lives of my peers. While the others all had houses to go home to each night, we did not. Every day, the three of us would stay late after school until about six o'clock. Once we were convinced everyone had gone home, we would sneak out to get something small for dinner. When we returned to the empty school, we would take out our mattresses and pillows from where we kept them hidden, push the chairs to the side and then sleep on the floor. Each morning, we took a bath, ironed our clothes and were always the first ones at school — because we never really left.

I grew to love Dad very much, but I must admit, he was a demanding taskmaster and a disciplinarian, who could be very soldier-like in his ways. For example, when he would go out to tutor a student to earn extra money, he would always leave something for my brother and me to study while he was gone. When he returned, he would expect us to recite what we learned. To this day, the words of William Shakespeare, Winston Churchill and other famous orators remain with me.

Although he could be strict, Dad made sure we never doubted his love for us. Most of the time, he was both our mother and our father. People in our town called us the Three Musketeers because we were always together. He took us to the market to get what we needed. He taught school to earn money to support us. And he was also the one who cooked for us. He never owned a car or a house because he always invested everything he had into our educations.

The importance of achieving a good formal education is only part of the values my father instilled in us. I am a doctor today and love taking care of people because of the love that my father displayed for all forms of life. One time, we saw some baby chicks in a ditch without a mother hen in sight. Dad worried that if it rained, the chicks would drown, so he had my brother and me go on either side of the ditch to round up the chicks. He then looked for the chicks' home and made sure they were safe.

I remember on more than one occasion coming across someone in the street who was not right in the head. My father had no extra money to give these people, but he would walk to wherever we were living, find some of his own clothes and bring them back for the person. And if we could not locate them – even after a long search – Dad would leave the clothes for the person to find. Looking back, I can recall seeing several homeless people in our city wearing my father's clothes over the years.

He told my brother and me: "If I never have many material possessions, as long as I give you both a good education and a love of God, I will be happy."

4

Mom, Dad ... And Maureen

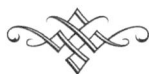

Sandra Lee Pope was born in Napa, California. Because of her father's job as an electrician, her family moved around a lot when she was young. They eventually settled in Placerville – a Northern California town of about 10,000 as famous for its proximity to Sutter's Mill where gold was discovered in 1848 as it is infamous for being known back in the day as "Hangtown."

Mom was a beautiful young woman with a strong personality whose need to always be right wouldn't allow her to shy away from a good argument, even with a complete stranger. She was tall and slender with straight brown hair, lovely teeth, and the kind of full lips that women these days pay a lot of money to have created for them. When Mom was 19 and her sister, Marsha, was 16, their mother died from a brain hemorrhage at age 45. Then when her father started drinking heavily, she knew she couldn't stay.

As near as I can tell, it was at about the time Mom's family was falling apart that her mental well-being began to unravel as well. I can't help but think that all this trauma and loss at an early age was part of the reason she was always searching for someone or something to fix her broken heart. Ultimately, she moved to San Francisco.

The 1960s were an exciting time for an impressionable teenager to be living on her own in a city awash in counterculture. She met Donald

Edward Pope in a bar and six weeks later they married. Not long after that, my brother Eddie was born. My parents wanted more children, but after six years of trying, it still hadn't happened. Mom suffered from endometriosis, and they thought she wasn't going to get pregnant again, so they took in a foster infant, my sister Jenny, with the intention of eventually adopting her. But, of course, fate stepped in and within a month Mom was pregnant with twins – my sister Stephanie and me.

I'm sure that suddenly going from having just one child to care for to seemingly overnight being responsible for raising four kids under age 10 took a toll on Mom and Dad's marriage. Dad had begun drinking more frequently and often left Mom on her own for days at a time, which meant she had to take care of three infant girls and a 7-year-old boy while he was away working for the railroad.

At some point, Mom had been diagnosed with clinical depression, so I'm sure being left on her own to raise four young kids couldn't have helped her mental state. Her frustration eventually grew so great over the situation that she kicked Dad out and let her friend Maureen and her kids move in. Maureen and Mom shared a bedroom, and my parents eventually divorced.

The first thing I can remember from my childhood is from when I was 4 years old. It was right around Valentine's Day when I woke up in the middle of the night and wandered into the living room where I found some of Maureen's heart candies. I had begun eating them, like any kid that age would have, when Maureen caught me. I saw the anger boiling in her eyes, and I can still feel the fear that consumed me that night many years ago just like it was yesterday. That is also the first time I can remember Maureen beating me.

Years later, when I asked Mom about that beating, she reacted like she always did when the topic of abusive behavior from our childhood came up.

"I never saw anything like that!" she would say without giving it a thought. "If that happened, it must have been when I wasn't there!"

Mom had her own abusive side as well. When I was little, I sucked my thumb for comfort. Determined to break me of this habit, Maureen began putting hot sauce on my fingers in an attempt to deter this behavior. I was also forced to lie on the floor just outside their bedroom door, so Mom and Maureen could make sure I didn't suck my thumb. I vividly recall the two of them laughing and refusing to give me water after I put my fingers that were coated in hot sauce in my mouth and started crying.

I have no idea when or why Maureen left our house, but thankfully she did. Eventually, my parents got back together. Dad moved back in, and they remarried and bought a house in Lincoln, California. Of course, that didn't last. They separated again three years later but never officially divorced.

The years that followed are a chaotic blur of random scenes of childhood memories. The more stressful life became, the more Mom began physically showing her age. By my middle school years, her hair was starting to gray and more wrinkles were taking up residence on her face.

Through all the chaos and upheaval, Dad was my constant. I always knew he loved us kids. He made sure to tell us that every chance he could. I stayed with him on weekends when he wasn't working, and I remember him crying once when he dropped us off at Mom's house after a weekend together. He knew how crazy our life with Mom was, and he felt bad he wasn't in a place to do anything about it.

Most of the time when I was young, we lived off child support, government loans and welfare. Mom would get jobs at places like Carl's Jr. and day care centers, but those never lasted. She always said or did something to put her foot in her mouth and that job would end. She just couldn't seem to keep her mouth shut or her bizarre opinions to herself.

Mom was always taking college classes and after probably more than a decade she finally earned a degree. As a student, she qualified for financial assistance, and I'm sure she never repaid these loans. I'm guessing that when Mom died, she probably owed the government well over $100,000 in student loans.

Even though she was well-educated and loved teaching children, Mom never really held a job. At one point after she finished school, she was a substitute teacher. I remember the day she subbed at my high school – I was mortified. She had no classroom management skills and spoke in a degrading manner to students, including a couple of my friends.

Needless to say, she didn't get asked back.

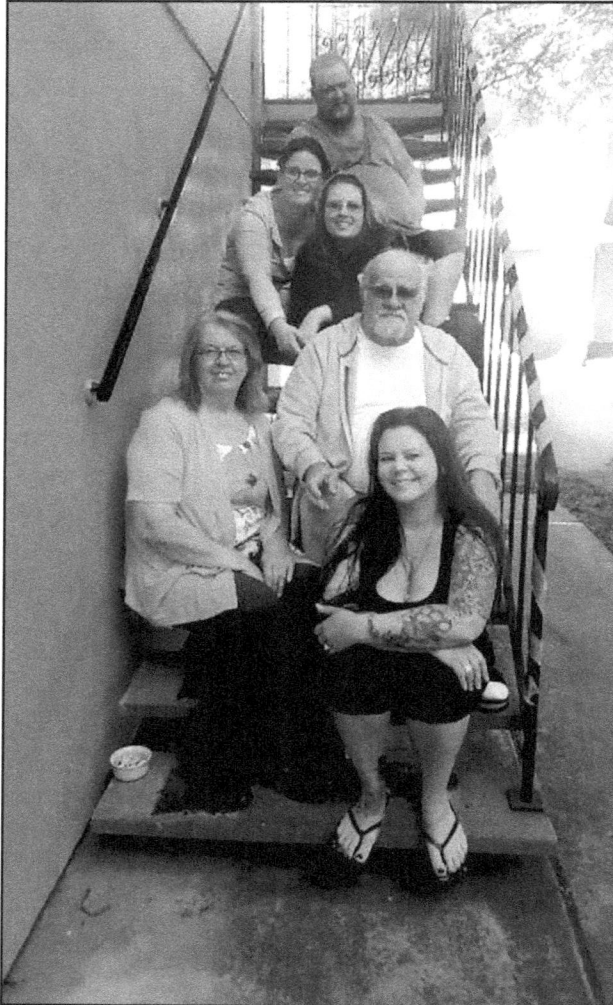

5

Fear Of Fire

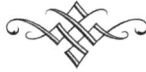

I've always had an irrational fear of fire. When I go camping, I must check and recheck that the campfire is out before I can go tosleep. Even something as silly as the barbeque grill in our backyard causes me irrational concern. Several times over the years, I have woken up drenched in sweat after a nightmare involving either myself or my loved ones who are trapped in a fire.

Only recently have I been able to connect the dots between the neglect my mother showed all of us children growing up and how this anxiety about fire originally took control over me. The mystery began to unravel shortly after our Dad died in 2015. Eddie was at my house one day, and he started talking about a fire that happened when we were very young.

"What are you talking about?" I said. "What fire?"

"You know, when our house caught fire when we were kids," said Eddie, seven years my elder. "Mom never told you about that? I guess you were too young to remember."

"What the hell?" I said, feeling like I'd just been punched in the gut.

"It wasn't too long after Maureen (our neighbor) and her three kids moved in with us," Eddie began. "You and Stephanie must have been about 3, Jen must've been 4, and I was like 10.

"Something caught fire in the kitchen, and when I got outside, Mom and Maureen were just standing there in the front yard talking. I'm the one who asked where you girls were. It was like they had forgotten you were in the house. I went back in and got all three of you out. We made it to the backyard, but we couldn't get to the front because the heat was too intense.

"Thankfully, I heard a firefighter calling our names. He was able to get all of us to the front of the house with Mom and Maureen."

Tears welled up in Eddie's eyes as he recounted the details. This certainly explained my fear of fire, even though I had no recollection of the tragedy that could have killed all of us. Worse yet, I had *no* trouble believing Mom would have left us inside a burning house. To her, we were replaceable. She was always looking for a newer, better family that would accept her more freely and make her depression go away.

Throughout her entire life, Mom always thought the grass was greener somewhere else. That's why she and my father split when I was 3, and she let our lesbian neighbor and her kids move in. That's why she eventually remarried Dad and then left him a second time. That's why she moved in with Bill, her physically abusive boyfriend. And that is most certainly why later she lied to my face for eight months before secretly moving to Germany and then to Ghana.

She was always looking for someone or something that would miraculously make her life better. Eventually, that's why Mom left Germany and at age 66 moved to Africa to be with a man one-third her age that she met on the internet. In my heart, I know she kept seeking those greener pastures right up until she died as a result of that mysterious car crash.

6

Bad News Bill

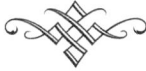

I was 9 the first time I met Bill, and more than 30 years later I still vividly remember the day we were introduced. We were living in the Lincoln house, and Mom was taking classes at a local junior college One day when I went to visit her, the two of us were sitting together on a bench when a man with long, dirty blonde hair, thick glasses and a filthy T-shirt walked up, and that was when Mom introduced me to Bill.

The two of us were sitting together on a bench when a man with long, dirty blonde hair, thick glasses and a dirty T-shirt walked up, and Mom introduced me to Bill. She said he was in one of her classes, but after he walked away, she continued making a big deal out of telling me how much he annoyed her. Even a kid could tell they were flirting. Sure enough, within a couple of weeks, Mom invited Bill to our house. She introduced him to all of us kids, and then, without warning, announced we would all be moving in with Bill and his two daughters.

Probably the lowest point of my roller coaster childhood was the time we spent living with Bill and his family. Bill's house was an old barn that had been converted into a small three-bedroom house where two adults and five girls shared one bathroom. Eddie had gotten into trouble and wasn't living with us at this point, so it was just my sisters and I who were displaced this time.

Bill had a temper and could be abusive. I was getting old enough to remember more details about the episodes of domestic violence that occurred, and my memories from that time are crystal clear. But just like with Maureen, Mom shut herself off from the harsh realities of domestic abuse, claiming never to have seen anything.

Bill doled out the discipline with an iron fist, and Mom was more than happy to let him do it. When my sisters or I were in trouble, Mom would wait until Bill got home to punish us because she said, "he can hit harder." Mom was right about that. On more than one occasion, I felt firsthand just how much harder.

One day when I was 12, my sisters and I had been across the street at a friend's house playing, and when we got home, Bill was upset at Jenny for not doing a chore he had told her to do. I was sitting next to Mom on the couch. I remember Jenny staring at him with a look of fear mixed with the blank stare of a deer caught in the headlights. Bill became enraged and started yelling. It was clear he was about to get physically abusive.

That's when I finally snapped. "Fuck this!" I yelled at Mom as I got in between Bill and Jenny. "You're not our father, and you have no right to touch us!" I screamed in his face.

My memories of the next few minutes are kind of fuzzy. Bill's hands flew around my throat, and he began choking me and screaming obscenities as he pushed me into a corner of the room. I was starting to black out when Mom finally pulled Bill off me. I'm not sure who called the police, but they showed up that night. It was one of the scariest moments of my life, but I would do it again because that was the night we finally broke free from Bill.

Even before the time when I stood up to Bill, I had already moved out of his house and in with Aunt Marsha because I needed to go to a school that would help me with my learning disabilities. Aunt Marsha was my Mom's younger sister, but she definitely was the more responsible one of the two. The sisters had an on-again, off-again relationship, and there were years they didn't speak to each other.

During all the random moving around we did throughout my

childhood, the one place where I could find refuge and stability was Aunt Marsha's house. She had always wanted a girl, and as a result we were very close. She treated me like one of her own children, and for the first time in my life, I really felt the parental love that I never did from my own Mom. Marsha made sure that we were clean and fed – something that never worried Mom – and she took us to church. Aunt Marsha had a pool, so we kids loved going there. I was so happy there, but in my heart, I knew this couldn't last.

After my fight with Bill, Mom, Jenny and Stephanie also moved in with Aunt Marsha. The arrangement was doomed from the start. Mom was a chain smoker, and that caused friction right off the bat. One day I was sitting in the front room and heard Mom and Marsha arguing in the kitchen. When I heard the first dish break, I silently prayed that it had been an accident. When I heard the second, third and who knows how many more plates hitting the floor, all I could do was cry. Without a word being spoken, I knew we would have to leave.

From then on, the two sisters seldom uttered a word to one another. Mom would need something, or Aunt Marsha would feel guilty, and so they would get back in touch. The last time they ever spoke was shortly after their dad died. Somehow, in my grandfather's will, one of them ended up receiving about $1,000 more than the other. I honestly don't remember which one, but that $1,000 dollars caused such hard feelings that the sisters never reconciled. Mom and Aunt Marsha died six weeks apart without ever speaking to each other again.

7

(Alfred)
A Test From God ... Or The Devil

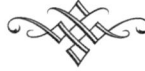

As a teacher of English and mathematics, my father firmly believed education was the path to a better future. Many of the students who passed through his hands went on to successful careers, and he mentored several pupils who won awards in international writing competitions. They would tell me stories about how my Dad influenced their lives, and on more than one occasion someone would ask, "Are you Mr. Aidoo's son?" "Yes, I am lucky enough to be his son," I would tell them.

In Ghana, teaching is a respected profession, but it does not pay a lot of money. When times were good, we had enough money to rent a house, but we were also evicted a couple of times when we could not pay the rent. At times we lived with family members, but that could be frustrating for us and for them. My Dad helped anyone he could, and just like my father, there isn't a person I would not help. When I see someone in pain, I can tell by their actions if not their words, that they need help. And I have the God-given ability to gain the trust of people who need love and support and make them feel that someone cares about them. I can do this because I know how it feels to go through challenges without much support. I do whatever I can to help people who are suffering. This is why I am a doctor.

Constantly witnessing so many human frailties on a daily basis taught me compassion and empathy, but it also has taken a toll on my physical, mental and emotional health. I sometimes become depressed by all the human suffering I see and my inability to provide more help. The struggles of those around me eventually become my burden as well. That is just the way my soul has formed. I care about other people, and I find myself sinking into sadness at times. These are the times when God is testing me.

When I feel this sadness, I often go to a botanical reserve and spend hours just looking at the trees and thinking about the lives of people around me. I know these times of solitude have taken me away from friends and family, but it is important to me to keep my sadness to myself. When I was in medical school, there were times when I played the role of the happy friend who could make everyone laugh, and then afterward I would go home and cry because I felt like there was nobody there for me. When these dark moods came upon me, I could not see a future for myself. Sometimes I thought life was futile.

As a doctor I have been blessed to help many people over the years. Knowing what I do now with the benefit of experience, I know the futility I felt and continue to sometimes feel is either a test from God or a challenge from God's adversary — maybe both. Despite all these challenges, I believe that through the grace of God and the teachings of my father, I have been fortunate to become an instrument in God's hand. Without His divine guidance, I would have never become a doctor.

Medical school was not easy. It was hard studying alongside students whose only concern was passing their classes, while in addition to my studies I had to worry about where my next meal was coming from. For about two months I was penniless and would have starved if not for the kindness of my roommate who shared his meals with me. But I was in no position to complain. While at least I had a roof over my head, my father was frequently homeless because any extra money he made he would send to help get me through school.

By the grace of God, I graduated in 2007 and began my internship (or housemanship as we call it in Ghana) in trauma orthopedics at Komfo Anokye Teaching Hospital in Kumasi. After two years, I was done with my schooling. I hoped to be hired as a medical officer at the teaching hospital, but when I didn't hear anything right away, I decided to keep working until I did.

"You're crazy!" a friend said. "Your housemanship is over. What if you do all this extra work, and they decide not to hire you?"

"At least I will keep acquiring experience and continue helping people," I said.

Thankfully, I was hired as a medical officer. My boss was happy enough with my work that he wrote letters on my behalf to the hospital management and even to the Ghanaian Ministry of Health. I worked in that job for seven years, and eventually there was little I couldn't do in the department. More importantly, this was where I really developed my philosophy that we need to not only treat our patients but their families as well.

One day a lady came into the emergency room with a crushed leg. As I started treating her, I noticed a man standing in the corner looking very worried. As soon as I had a minute to talk to him, I learned that he was the lady's husband, and he was scared for her life. I comforted him as much as I could and promised to do everything I could to heal her. We got her into the operating room quickly and repaired her damaged leg.

Years later, I saw the man and even though a long time had passed since we had seen each other, he went to great lengths to express how grateful he was for the care I had given both him and his wife. I find this effort to connect with our patients' families sorely lacking in our medical training. Of course, our primary responsibility is caring for our patients, but their family members are suffering too as they watch a loved one go through so much agony. How many times have you heard a parent say they would willingly take their child's pain on themselves if it were possible?

Even when people lose a loved one, they are comforted knowing that there is someone who cares about what they are going through. I get emotionally involved with my patients. I shed tears along with the families when a patient dies. I see allowing oneself to be this vulnerable in front of patients and families as an act of human kindness that is a strength, not as a sign of weakness or frailty. However, part of me knows it's a good thing for a doctor to stay emotionally distant from their patients because sharing the pain and agony of others can be a heavy burden. But quite honestly, I don't know any other way to care for people.

8

Man Plans; God Laughs

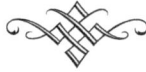

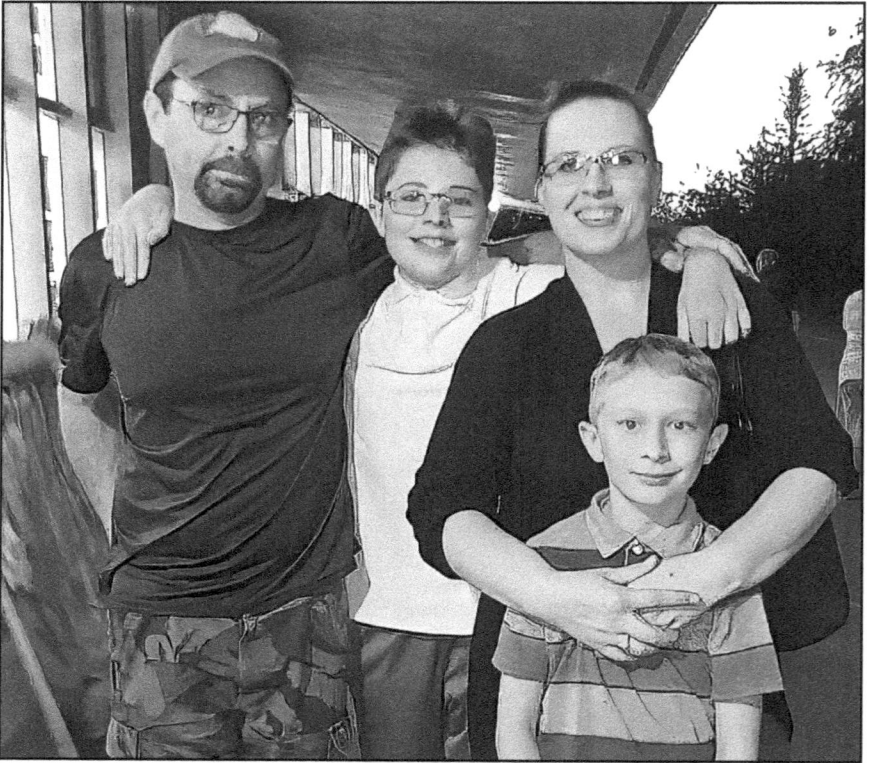

Katie's family

Eventually, I found a degree of normalcy among a group of friends at Oakmont High School in Roseville, California. Of course, just as my life was starting to settle into some sort of routine, Mom decided it was time to explore greener pastures once again. From out of nowhere she announced we were moving seven hours away to Crescent City on the California coast near the Oregon border.

No way was I going to let her pull me away from my friends before my senior year. I had finally been in the same school for three years in a row after attending five or six different elementary schools. I wanted to finish my senior year with my friends. Besides I was close enough in age to being an adult that Mom realized she couldn't force me to move. Plus, Dad still lived in Roseville, so I had a place to stay.

I honestly believe breaking away from Mom was the best decision I ever made because it allowed me to become the person I am today. My memories from those two years living with just my Dad are some of the sweetest of my life. He expected me to do my schoolwork and cared about my grades. Before this, I never realized the comfort that comes from having someone who cares about you set expectations and boundaries. I only wish I had this sort of structure when I was younger.

Eventually, Dad confided in me all the guilt he felt about not being able to take my siblings and me away from Mom sooner. He knew what a toll living with her was taking on his children, but his work schedule just wouldn't allow him to be a single parent for three kids.

I was the first child in my family to graduate high school. And by that time, I was already holding down two jobs, including one at the grocery store where I still work. Mom and the rest of the family came down for my graduation. Looking back, I am glad she came. But having Dad there was really the most important thing to me. I would not have succeeded without him, and he was so proud of me.

It came as no surprise when things didn't work out in Crescent City. After about two years Mom was back in town. By that point, I really didn't care where she was. I had carved out my own life, and frankly we hadn't been in contact much while she was gone. I just kept living my life without seeing much of her. Even my getting married didn't change things in any substantial way.

I met my husband, Rob, in 2002 while working as an assistant deli manager at a grocery store in Fair Oaks, California. Rob had transferred to the store as a head clerk, but neither of us really noticed the other in the first few weeks. When I worked in the deli, I had to keep my hair covered, so I usually wore a hat.

One day after work, I needed groceries, so I used one of the check-out aisles. Rob says he saw "my beautiful hair" for the first time from about four aisles away — and he was smitten. He asked me to lunch not long after that, but I turned him down. I was still on-again, off-again with my high school sweetheart, and besides, I really didn't want to get involved with someone at work. "That was the first time you made me feel stupid," Rob told me later.

We got to know each other better over the next few months, so when he asked me again to have lunch, I considered it. I honestly didn't have time that day, so I said maybe another time. Unfortunately, that was the same day my ex-boyfriend showed up unannounced at work. He owed me rent money, so I had to meet him on my break. We were sitting in front of a Baskin-Robbins near the store when Rob happened by at the end of his lunch break. Seeing me there with another guy after I told him I didn't have time to have lunch with him didn't just look bad, it was bad. Things were falling apart before they even had a chance to begin. After that, Rob didn't speak to me for six months. He told me later that was the second time I made him feel stupid.

Months later, Sarah, my best friend from high school who worked in the bakery, invited me over for dinner one evening. She was married, but it wasn't unusual for me to hang out with her and her husband, so I didn't think anything about the invite. When Rob approached me at work later that day and said, "I hear we're having dinner together tonight," I was shocked. "What are you talking about?" I said, totally unaware that we were being set up.

Apparently, that was strike three. I had made Rob feel stupid again. In my defense, I really didn't know what he was talking about. Sarah later admitted she had set the whole thing up because she thought Rob was perfect for me. Rob and I hit it off. In some ways, he reminded me of my Dad. He was sweet and confident. His infectious laugh really won me over. We started dating, and about nine months later, I moved in with him.

Unlike me, Rob had pretty much lived in the same house his whole life. His mom, Melva, owned a duplex with a smaller two-bedroom, one-bath unit attached to a larger three-bedroom, two-bath home. Rob's parents divorced when he was young. At first, he lived with his mom in the larger part of the house but eventually moved into his own space in the smaller unit. Rob and his mom were remarkably close, and when she had a health scare with a pulmonary issue, it solidified his decision to stay nearby.

I came home from work one day not long after I moved in to find a nice dinner waiting in our kitchen. I knew Rob was at work, so it took me a minute to realize that Melva was the one who had left the dinner for us. I was confused, so I called Rob. "Do I owe your mom money for dinner?" I asked. "No," he laughed. "She does stuff like that all the time. She likes doing it."

Given my upbringing, that was so foreign to me. A gesture like that was something my own Mom would have never done. I didn't know how to react. Over time I grew to love having Rob's mom next door. She gave us our space but was always there for anything we needed. I really felt like I had a home for the first time since I had moved out of my Dad's house. Rob proposed to me on October 26, 2003, and I said yes without a second thought.

For about 10 years, I had been living my life without my Mom. She helped with my siblings' children, and I would see her occasionally at my sister's house, but we never made plans to specifically see each other.

Of course, I told my Mom about getting engaged thinking it might help us reconnect. She showed no signs of interest in helping me plan the wedding. Instead, it was Rob's mom who stepped in and did almost all the wedding planning and preparation with me. We made plans together and would go shopping. Quite often she would surprise me by completing some of the wedding details, so I didn't have to worry about everything. Just as an example, one day when I came home from work, I discovered she had bought all the favors for the bridesmaids.

When I asked my Mom for help, she chipped in $800 for the flowers, but that was it. About a month before the ceremony, we realized Mom still didn't have a dress, so Rob's mom went out and bought her a dress the same colors as her own. If it hadn't been clear before, it became abundantly apparent to me during the run-up to the wedding which woman really thought of me as a daughter.

On my wedding day, Mom was there physically at the ceremony but definitely not mentally. She was preoccupied with taking care of my sister's baby. She also was feuding with Aunt Marsha about not letting her hold the baby. I could tell that Rob's mom was irritated for my sake. I told her just to ignore the whole drama, so we could enjoy the wedding. "It is what it is," I told Melva.

When Rob and I got back from our honeymoon, Melva made a special lunch for us as we opened all the gifts from the wedding. Not surprisingly, Mom was invited but didn't make it. When we finished opening the last of the cards, it dawned on us that there was nothing from my Mom – not even a note wishing us well. I would have cherished a note from my Mom on my wedding day and kept it forever. I could tell by the look on Melva's face that she was heartbroken for me. In the time we had together, she did her best to be the mother I never had, and I loved her for that.

Rob and I decided to have kids right away because he is almost 10 years older than me. He was 37 when we got married and didn't want to be too old as a Dad to enjoy his children. Within three months, I was pregnant, and Melva was almost as excited as Rob and me. She had recently retired and was planning to watch the baby for us so that we wouldn't have to pay for day care. Once again, I was grateful for having such a loving mother-in-law next door.

About three months before my due date, Rob and I decided to take a mini vacation to Fort Bragg before I got too big to travel comfortably. We knew that it would probably be our last excursion without kids, so we drove three- and-half hours to the coast for a long-weekend getaway. We stopped in to say goodbye to Melva before we left, and we could both tell that she wasn't feeling well. She said she was just tired and insisted we go on our trip. When we said goodbye, she was cooking corned beef for dinner. There was no way to know it would be our last conversation.

The next evening while we were in Fort Bragg, Rob got a call from his sister, Jennifer. She had called their mom but hadn't been able to get ahold of her. Jennifer lived in Orinda, about an hour's drive from their mom, and she and Rob agreed that there wasn't anything to worry about just yet. We knew Melva liked to drink, and they thought that maybe she was either out with friends or had gone to bed early. The next day when Jennifer still couldn't contact her, they started to worry. Rob's friend Tracy lived across the street from the duplex, so Rob called and asked him to check on Melva.

Rob and Tracy were on the phone together as Tracy opened the unlocked front door of Melva's house. He immediately smelled the scorched corned beef on the stove and saw Melva's purse and keys on the table. Sensing something was wrong, Tracy told Rob he didn't see his mom but would call him back. Tracy found Melva's cold body on the bathroom floor. She had suffered a massive heart attack not long after we had said goodbye two days earlier.

When Tracy did not call Rob back immediately and was not answering Rob's calls, I sensed something wasn't right. So, I started packing our bags to go home. Rob called his Dad, who was still on friendly terms with his ex-wife even though they had been divorced for close to 40 years. Eventually, it was his Dad who broke the sad news to Rob that his mother was gone.

Rob collapsed when he heard what had happened. He was so stunned that the only words he could get out were, "She is never going to meet our baby." My heart was broken as well, but I knew I had to do my best to comfort Rob on our long solemn drive home. He was devastated.

Rob couldn't bring himself to live in the house anymore, and within a few months of his mom's passing, he and his sister sold the duplex. With our first baby on the way, Jennifer really helped us out by giving up her half of the inheritance to make sure that Rob and I could buy a house in the nice middle- class suburb of Fair Oaks. This simply would not have been possible on our salaries.

I felt lucky to have a new home, but I was also anxious about the move and the baby. We moved into the house on July 14, 2005, and Ryder was born September 5. While this was an exciting time for us, in some ways I felt like I was alone. Rob was present physically, but mentally he was lost in the deep emotional fog of grief as he mourned his mother's tragic passing.

Before long, I was drowning. I was juggling the stress of being a first-time mom caring for a newborn, with a heavy dose of guilt about getting back to work to keep our family afloat financially. Before her death, Rob's mom had planned to watch the baby while we worked, but now I had to find another solution. I looked into day care, but I just didn't make enough to offset the expense.

One solution kept staring me in the face, but I cringed every time I thought about it. Although I had been trying for years to distance myself from my Mom, she now had the one thing that we desperately needed. After years of going to school, Mom had at least one college degree, and she had experience working in childcare. While those who knew her best might have questioned her qualifications, the state of California saw fit to grant her a license to open an in-home day care center.

Asking Mom to include Ryder in her day care so I could continue to work seemed to be the most likely solution. But Mom had never really been a mother to me, and something inside of me fought to keep my child away from her. But I couldn't see any other way we could keep our house. Rob's mom and sister had sacrificed so much so that we could raise our family in a nicer neighborhood, so I felt like I owed them something. In the end, what else could I do? I swallowed my pride and called Mom.

Mom did OK as a day care provider. It was her business after all, and she had to maintain a level of professionalism to keep the doors open. Ryder was safe and we had free day care, but it came at a steep price. I was relying on the one person I would have preferred not to owe anything to.

A few years later when Mason was born, Mom was our salvation yet again. She now was the grandma who watched both our children. It was a role Rob and I dearly hoped his mother would fill. It's funny how life takes us in many directions we had never intended. Even though this was a path I never would have chosen, it led us exactly where we needed to be at the time. What is it they say, man plans, and God laughs?

9

(Alfred)
Alfred's Family

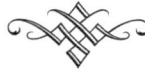

During my time at the University of Science and Technology in Kumasi, I became a campus elder in Lighthouse Chapel International where my roommate, Julian, was a pastor. Julian introduced me to his friend C. She was a shepherd in the church and lived in the apartment building next to ours and was studying forestry and renewable natural resources at the university.

Sometimes, after we came home from church meetings, C would prepare food and bring it over to Julian and me. At the time, all of us were so busy with our studies and serving in the church, it didn't occur to me to ask this beautiful, kind and caring person out on a date. That all changed, however, when I started my clinical rotations at the hospital and moved about 30 minutes away. It didn't take me long to realize that I missed seeing C. I missed our chats after church. That's when I made up my mind to get to know her better.

Eventually, we started dating. It wasn't always easy to see each other. Quite often I was bone tired after my clinical duties, but I would pay for a bus or taxi because I wanted to see her anytime I could. The bus dropped me off at the main gate of the campus, but it was still quite a walk to get to the residence hall where C lived – especially for a tired doctor in residence. No matter, as long as I could see C, even for a brief while, I didn't care how tired I was or if mosquitoes were eating me alive.

I have many fond memories from those days, but one particular trip to see C always brings a smile to my face. After getting off the bus at my usual stop, I had walked most of the way to her residence hall before she messaged me that she wasn't feeling well. So instead of visiting her right away, I went to the pharmacy and got her medicine. By the time I had walked all the way back to her apartment, I only had enough time to quickly drop off the medicine with her and head back to the hospital.

I was in love, and that is what love can make us do. Little could I have known that our chance meeting in college would blossom into a life-changing partnership? C and I got married in 2009 but decided that we wanted a little time to ourselves to get to know each other better before having children.

We welcomed our first beautiful daughter into our family in 2011, and three years later her sister joined us. We are not sure yet if we will have another child, but either way, I am a blessed and happy man.

The prevailing attitude for most men throughout Africa is to want sons to ensure that their family name carries on. For example, around the time our younger daughter was born, my mechanic friend was servicing the air conditioner in my car when suddenly he asked, "Alfred, has your wife given birth yet?"

I knew what he was getting at, but to prove a point and maybe change his attitude a little, I decided to be coy in my response.

"Yes, she did," I answered. "What did she have?" he asked.

"What do you mean, she had a baby," I said. "Boy or girl?" he snapped. "We had a second beautiful daughter," I told him proudly.

"You and I have the same problem," he confided.

"What problem is that?" I asked, continuing to lead him on.

"I also have two girls," he shared.

"When is having two beautiful and healthy girls ever a problem? I am a *proud* father of two girls," I replied.

Obviously, I have a different attitude than most African men. I'm not concerned whether my children are boys or girls. I am just happy that God has blessed C and me with two beautiful, healthy children to look after, and we try to give them the best lives possible. I just want my girls to be happy.

Like any family, we have had our ups and downs, and our lives can be hectic. C takes care of our girls, and she also works part-time as a field supervisor in community health in a Johns Hopkins' program that is supported by the Bill and Melinda Gates Foundation. C is very proud to be a part of this work, and I am proud of her as well.

As for me, I also find myself constantly balancing family life, my job and projects at the hospital, along with an ever-increasing role in serving the church. In 2005, I became a pastor and seven years later I was ordained as a reverend minister. I have been involved in overseeing multiple branches of our church as well as helping to train new shepherds and pastors.

Being together brings our family extraordinary joy, but we also love serving others. Although we are all pulled in many directions, God gives us the strength to do everything that He asks.

10

Down The Rabbit Hole

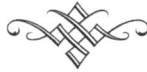

Dad was always loving and kind to people, even if they may not have deserved it. Because my parents never officially divorced, Mom was entitled to half of Dad's retirement income, which she gladly took. I was annoyed on his behalf, but Dad was OK with it. I think he could have cut her off anytime he chose, but that's not the kind of person Dad was. He knew Mom's personality had been poisoned by her mental illness. Plus, she had been his wife and was the mother of his children, so he felt responsible for her wellbeing.

Once Mom was able to collect part of Dad's retirement, she had enough money to live on, so she decided to close her day care. Ryder was five and Mason was two, and Mom watched them in her apartment for the next three years on days when Rob and I both worked. Mom and I still had our issues, but I'm forever grateful for her help during this time.

In 2013, my 18-year-old niece, Angelina, convinced Mom to move into an apartment with her to help pay the bills. Even though I had strongly advised Mom and Angelina against this living arrangement, my boys and I wound up being the ones who helped Mom move all her belongings into the apartment. Not surprisingly, in less than six weeks, this new living arrangement had failed. Angelina went her way and Mom moved in with us. While I was not disappointed with either

Angelina or Mom for the way things worked out in the end, I was, however, angry with my siblings since none of them showed up to help move Mom out of the apartment and into my house.

It was around this time, that Mom came out of our guest bedroom in tears, saying she had failed Angelina and wanted to kill herself. While this announcement was shocking on the surface, it lost a little of its luster because it wasn't the first time she had made this proclamation to me. But something felt different this time. Something was just a bit off about her behavior.

My concern quickly turned to anger, however, when I realized *what* the rant was really all about. I was deeply hurt by the words she chose to use that day.

"Why was Angelina so different that she was worth dying for?" I asked myself. "*WHAT ABOUT ME? WHY DIDN'T YOU CARE LIKE THIS ABOUT ME WHILE I WAS GROWING UP? WHAT ABOUT MY KIDS? AREN'T MY BOYS WORTH LIVING FOR?*"

I wanted to scream and slap Mom back into reality while she sat there selfishly ruminating over her desire to kill herself. Deep down I knew these were not the kind of things you say or actions you take when dealing with a suicidal person. Maybe seeing firsthand the kind of person Mom had become pushed me toward not ending up that selfish and petty. No matter how poorly she treated me, she was still my Mom, and part of me just couldn't turn my back on the woman who had given me life.

Thanks to Rob's sister, we have a nice, big house with an extra bedroom and bathroom that are removed from the rest of the house, so it was the perfect place for a long-term guest. Mom needed a place to stay, and we still needed someone to watch the boys after school when Rob and I both worked, so of course it made sense to let her move in.

But the idea of living under the same roof as my mother tore me up inside. I knew the kind of mother she had been to me – or more accurately, that she had *not* been a mother at all. It scared me to think of the kinds of things I might be exposing my own children to with her around 24-7. Still, having Mom watch them at her place had turned out OK. But I knew having her live at our house full-time would be different. Plus, I knew it would be tough on our marriage.

If the arrangement with Mom was going to have any hope of working, there would have to be ground rules – not the least of which was religiously keeping her on her medications. Mom had a history of starting on antidepressants, but she would never stay on them for long. I made it very clear to Mom that before she could move in with us, she had to commit to seeing a mental health doctor on a regular basis. I also insisted that she take any medication the doctor prescribed.

I am quite sure there were other issues at work in my mother's mental state besides depression – probably bipolar or other personality disorders – but she never received any other diagnoses. It wasn't for lack of trying on the part of doctors. Mom had been diagnosed with clinical depression, but when doctors had suggested more tests to get a better picture of her psyche, Mom had always refused. Maybe something inside her didn't want to know the truth because it might disrupt her existence.

Despite all the bitterness between Mom and me, something inside told me there was still hope that things would get better this time. Mom saw this as yet another chance to start over again with me, so she agreed to my terms. If Mom could stay on her meds, maybe *this time* would be different. I desperately needed a *real* mom. So much so that I fantasized about the two of us laughing and talking on the couch like a normal mother and daughter.

Perhaps, at first, I only saw what my heart was aching to see, because it seemed like my dream of a normal loving and caring mom was becoming a reality. She appeared better, and for the first time I could remember since I was a kid, she and I truly laughed together.

In some ways this glimmer of hope made it even more painful when things came crashing down around us – and they did collapse, all too quickly.

In the beginning, Mom helped watch the boys and picked them up from school. Her living with us made things more convenient. So much so, that even Rob, who normally doesn't get along well with my family, was supportive of her being there. That all ceased abruptly when Mom discovered the internet.

Mom always had an obsessive personality. The earliest examples always involved religion. She would become totally sold on a particular brand of religion for a few months or even a year, but eventually someone or something would set her off, and she would find another church. I have fond memories of the nice people in some of these congregations, but I also recall experiences that I would call "crazy churches."

After we were adults, Eddie and I would talk about this period of our childhood. When I'd say "crazy finds crazy" we would both laugh because each of us knew exactly what I meant.

For most of my adult life, I have been turned off by organized religion. Only recently, with Alfred's help, have I begun to understand that I really do believe in God. I am starting to see a plan for my life that I must admit is guided by a higher power.

Mom also obsessed about her hobbies like sewing, quilting and writing. She would become fixated with something for a while, tire of it and then move on. Foolishly, I assumed that's how it would be with the internet. But I was wrong. As her screen time increased with online chats and gaming with friends she met in cyberspace, I watched her slowly disappear into the darkness of the web.

The World Wide Web became Mom's *ultimate* addiction. Once this digital drug grabbed her, she was unable to break free. In hindsight, it makes sense that a rabbit hole filled with the world's collective knowledge, images and boundless ideas would be too much temptation for someone with a compulsive personality like Mom. Especially one who always has one eye trained on finding greener pastures.

At first, Mom just chatted with random people from around the world using her cellphone. From there things escalated quickly. She bought her first tablet to make it easier to keep in contact with her new friends.

When she became particularly close with some people in Germany, she would set an alarm to wake up in the middle of the night and go online to chat and game with them when they were awake. Her sleep pattern completely turned upside down, Mom compensated by taking naps during the day. But those catnaps gave way to Mom sleeping the entire day. This meant she was no longer helping to watch the boys, so she was failing the primary purpose we had for her living in our house.

11

Your Damn Boys

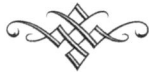

With Mom either sleeping or chatting online all the time, Rob had reached his breaking point with her. There was a stretch when she pretty much stayed in her room playing on the internet, and Rob stayed in our bedroom across the house because he didn't want to see her. I was stuck in the middle unable to make either of them happy but trying my best to take care of the boys.

Things came to a head one evening. Rob and I were both working, and when I called home to check on things, Ryder told me they hadn't eaten dinner because Grandma had been asleep since they had gotten home from school that afternoon.

I was none too happy about that revelation, but it got much worse when I got home from work that night, and Mom greeted me with, "One of your damn boys cut the cord!"

"What are you talking about?" I said.

"Those boys broke the internet cord!" she screamed. That was the moment I realized just how dependent Mom had become on the internet. Somehow while the boys were playing earlier that day the router had been damaged, resulting in our Wi-Fi going out. Mom was beside herself with anger that night when I got home from work. I had never seen her so upset with the boys. I was so frustrated with her that I just walked away without saying anything.

Later that night I found her sitting in my car in front of the house. "I'm staying out here, because your damn internet is out," she informed me when I went to check on her.

"Mom, it's after midnight," I said.

"I don't care," she said, "this is where I get the best reception on my cellphone."

Again, I just walked away shaking my head. I had no energy to fight with her. She stayed in the car talking to her friends online for a couple of hours in the middle of the night burning through cellular data time because our Wi-Fi was out.

After she had gotten a few hours of sleep, Mom drove to Eddie's and demanded he help her find the right cable to "fix the internet at Katie's house because her boys had broken it." Eddie helped her buy a new cord, and Mom was right back talking to her friends again that night.

We were all mentally and emotionally drained by the living situation. Mom was no longer pitching in to help with the boys, but I was hesitant to bring it up with her because I could see that she was spiraling into depression. I asked her a few times if she was happy. All she would say was, "it's just different living here instead of in my own place." But I saw through her façade. I knew she wasn't happy.

Mom had been living with us for about a year when she told me in late 2014 that she was planning a trip to get together with some of the people she had met online. She and her friends from Germany were going to spend three weeks together in Virginia. She said they were meeting at the end of November and would stay together through Christmas. It seemed strange that none of her friends wanted to be near their families during the holidays. But oddly, in a way it was a bit of a relief. Maybe the trip would boost her mood and lift her spirits.

I believed that a break from each other after a year of living under the same roof would be a good thing. After living with us rent free while collecting half of Dad's retirement, Mom had saved up a little money, so at first I supported the trip, but I got suspicious when Mom mentioned something about needing a passport.

"You don't need a passport to go to Virginia," I told her.

"I know," she said. "It's just in case I need it at some point."

That didn't sound like an honest answer, and my mind flashed back to the bit of conversation I overheard when she mentioned "a new life." Things in my mind were clicking into place, so I asked my mother directly, "Mom, are you coming back?"

"Yes, I am coming back," she said, dismissing my concern. "I would never leave without telling you. You're my daughter. I love you."

Despite all she said, I had a strange feeling about Mom's trip. We didn't see much of her the days before she left. Her sleep patterns were still off, and she spent more time packing than I expected. She packed some weird things for a three-week trip. She had a bunch of Cabbage Patch dolls that she had made clothes for when she was on her sewing kick, and she took several of those. That seemed strange, but I thought maybe she wanted to show off her sewing to her friends.

I thought that if she were really leaving for good, she would have at least wanted to spend a little time with us that day. She used her tablet to take a couple pictures of the boys. The next morning when I had to leave for work, Mom was in her room, and I thought about going in to say goodbye, but I was kind of irritated at her for not spending time with us the day before. Besides, I thought she would only be gone for a few weeks, so I went to work.

Jenny drove Mom to the airport, and as far as anyone knew, she was heading to Virginia. When an airport worker came to help Mom with her luggage, Jenny heard him mention something about Germany. Jenny was totally blindsided.

"Where are you really going, Mom?" she asked. "I have a one-way ticket to Germany," she finally admitted. "I'm never coming back, and I'm finally happy."

Jenny waited two weeks to break the news to me that Mom had gone to Germany. "Are you sitting down?" she asked over the phone, knowing full well I was about to start my 8 a.m. shift at work.

"No, why?" I said.

"Mom's in Germany. She says she's finally happy, and she's *not* coming back," Jenny said as I broke down in tears. "I thought that you would be happy that Mom is happy."

The funny thing is that looking back on the situation, Jenny was probably right about the whole thing. From a logical point of view, I should have been happy and relieved about Mom's departure. But my brain couldn't convince my heart – she was my Mom! She had abandoned me before, but this time my children got caught in her emotional wake. Foolishly, I had let her back into my life – into my boys' lives – so I only had myself to blame for being naïve enough to think this time would be different. Still, it stung when I thought about all the time I had wasted dealing with her ups and downs over the last year without any help from my siblings.

I was in a haze the rest of the day. Mom had looked me in the eye and lied to my face when I asked her directly if she was coming back. She played me for a fool, and then left me, again. Had the last year living with us been just a game to Mom? Did anyone matter to her?

When I finally got home from a long day, Dad was there watching the boys. I fell into him like I was 10 years old and wept. He cried with me. "I'm sorry she did this to you," he said. "You didn't deserve this. I love you." He stroked my hair, and I cried on his shoulder for 20 minutes before I went into the bathroom and threw up.

I realized then that I would never see or talk to Mom again. That was the first time I mourned for my mother.

12

The Bottom Falls Out Of My World

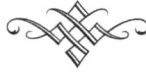

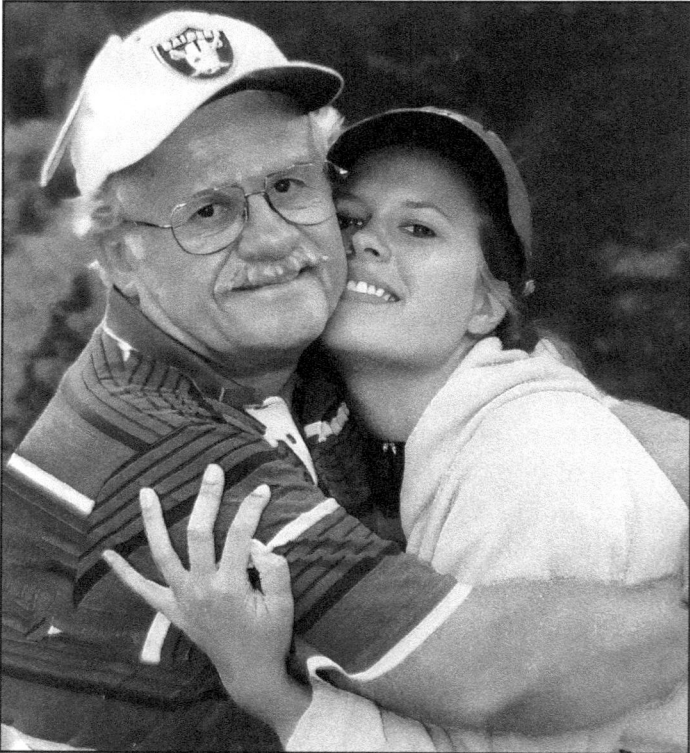

Katie and her father

The bottom fell out of my world on October 20, 2015. Rob and I had been arguing off and on for a while, so Dad offered to let the boys and me stay at his house anytime we needed. After a pretty bitter exchange with Rob on October. 19, I decided to take Dad up on his offer. I hesitated to call him because I wasn't sure if I was going to follow through with actually going there, and I didn't want to stress him out unnecessarily.

Eventually, I talked myself out of the idea because the boys had school the next day and I had work. I never told Dad how close I came to accepting his offer. To this day, I have mixed emotions about my decision.

I was at work the next morning when my sister Stephanie called. She was trying to say something, but no words were coming out. Eddie took the phone and his voice cracked as he said, "Dad is gone."

"What do you mean, Dad is gone?" I said. "Dad is dead," Eddie replied. "How do you know?" I asked, hoping it wasn't true.

"We just found him upstairs," my brother answered.

I collapsed onto the floor of the empty back room of the store. I sat on the ground for at least five minutes clutching the phone and hoping to hear something different from my brother. Of course, the news didn't change. I felt all alone.

I finally gathered myself enough to hang up the phone and try to find someone to tell that I was leaving. It felt like nobody cared. When I told my boss what had happened, he actually asked if I would be back the following day to write orders. "No," I told him and walked out the door.

I drove to Dad's house on autopilot. I just kept thinking, "Did he know how much I loved him? Was I a good enough daughter?" When I arrived, the sheriff wouldn't let me in because they had to make sure that no crime had been committed. "You don't want to see him like that, anyway," Eddie said.

Apparently, Dad had a heart attack on the couch and rigor mortis had set in. They couldn't lay him flat when the coroner wheeled his body out of the apartment two hours later. I couldn't bear to watch as they loaded him into the van and drove away. If only I had gone over to his house the night before, maybe I would have been able to do something, or at least tell him goodbye and how much I loved him. The coroner showed a lot of concern for us. "You're going to hurt as much as you loved him," she shared. I think about her words almost every day.

I was relieved that I hadn't told Dad about my argument with Rob because he was the kind of person who took on the pain of his children. I don't know if I could have lived with myself wondering if the stress of us coming to his house the night before had somehow contributed to his death. Losing my Dad was probably the worst day of my life. He was the parent who acted like a parent. He was an amazing man and so special to me. He loved me and my siblings unconditionally. He was my rock.

Jenny wanted to call Mom right away and tell her about Dad, but I begged her not to. By this time Mom had lived in Germany for almost a year, and what little news I got about her came from my sister and brother. Mom didn't have a lot of money but was somehow surviving on the $1,600 a month she got from Dad's retirement. Mom was dating people she met on websites and had managed to get into trouble with one boyfriend because she ran up his credit card without permission. Typical Mom.

"She does *not* care, Jenny!" I told my sister. "She won't come. ... She wants his money, and as soon as she knows he's dead, she'll take it all." But I've learned over the years that Jenny generally *does* what Jenny *wants*, so she called Mom anyway.

"*Here we go,*" I thought.

As hard as that day was for me, the next morning was worse. I woke up and for just a second, it felt like a normal day. Suddenly everything from the day before washed over me, and I felt like I was drowning, and I seriously didn't know what to do. I wanted the world to stop and mourn with me. If I had to hurt this much, it wasn't fair that other people were happy. I was even angry that the sun was shining. Fortunately, those feelings didn't last long. I began thinking about what Dad wanted for all of us, and I knew that I couldn't stay angry at the world for long. That would not be fair to his memory and his wishes.

I knew Dad wanted a simple memorial. He made the arrangements himself and prepaid for cremation, so the responsibility of planning his funeral wouldn't fall on any of us. But instead of Dad's wishes, Jenny arranged a big memorial service that included an open casket. Since he was being cremated, it meant we had to rent a casket for the viewing (I didn't even know that you could do something like that).

Of course, all of these changes would cost more money. Dad had set some funds aside, but Mom had frozen it all. Since they had never divorced and she was already collecting half of Dad's retirement, it was easy for her to call the Railroad Board and divert all of his money – just like I knew she would. She certainly wasn't going to pay for any part of Dad's funeral, even though it was his money.

We all told Jenny that her changes would cost too much money and, more importantly, her memorial service was not what Dad had expressed that he wanted. But Jenny's mind was made up, so we moved ahead with her plan.

Speaking at Dad's service really helped me work through some things. I talked about the gifts that he had given me. He was such a loving and amazing person. One of the things that he talked to me about was forgiveness.

He told me that I needed to forgive Mom for my own sake. He had taken Mom back after she left him for Maureen. Even after she left him for good, he had never legally divorced her. I'm sure he could have blocked her from taking half of his retirement, but he gave it to her willingly. Dad had found happiness in his life, and I realized that was the example I needed to follow. Although it wasn't going to be easy, and it wouldn't happen overnight, I too would have to find a way to forgive my mother.

I thought I would have a little time alone in Dad's house after he died to start going through his things. It helped me feel close to him. But within 30 minutes, Angelina started moving her things into Dad's part of the fourplex.

We had agreed as a family that she could move in at the end of the month, so I was unpleasantly surprised when Jenny let her daughter move into Dad's house the week he died. We hadn't even had a chance to sort through his belongings.

But even as irritated as I was about that, it was nothing compared to the anger I felt in the next three weeks. At some point, Angelina and Jenny realized that the monthly mortgage needed to be paid. Knowing that Mom had taken all of Dad's money, Angelina texted her to ask if they could use some of the money to cover the mortgage until we could get everything squared away. Mom texted back she didn't have the money.

Something inside me snapped when I saw that. I hadn't spoken with our mother in close to a year, but I grabbed Angelina's phone and sent her a scathing, expletive-filled text:

HOW DARE YOU? ALL YOU CARE ABOUT IS YOURSELF! WE ARE HERE MOURNING OUR DAD – MAKING FUNERAL ARRANGEMENTS AND SETTLING HIS AFFAIRS. YOU TOOK ALL OF HIS MONEY AND AREN'T HELPING WITH ANY OF HIS FUNERAL! EVERY TIME YOU SPEND A PENNY OF DAD'S MONEY, YOU'D BETTER THANK HIM BECAUSE WITHOUT HIM, YOU WOULD HAVE NOTHING! I WILL NEVER TALK TO YOU AGAIN!

Then I told her to "fuck off." That was the last thing I ever said to my mother that I knew she could understand.

13

Death Visits Us Again

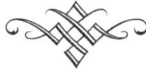

A few months before Dad died, I tried my hand at refinishing an old bed frame in the shabby-chic style using chalk paint. I really liked the look and decided that I wanted to try it for myself. My first attempt ended up with the bed frame looking like I had dipped it in Pepto-Bismol. But after watching several YouTube videos, I finally went into a shop called Not Too Shabby in Folsom. The shop owner, Bobbi, was wonderful, and she gave me the advice I needed to do it right.

I was able to lose myself in painting, and it became a way for me to feel creative and productive. Dad absolutely loved the furniture, and he encouraged me to try to sell some of the pieces, but I had no idea where to even start marketing something like this.

I displayed several of my furniture pieces alongside pictures of Dad at his reception at our house. I was proud that the display turned out well, and I knew Dad would have been happy, too. I received a lot of compliments on the picture galleries and the shabby-chic furniture. Several people asked where I had bought them, and when I told them that I had painted them myself, they wanted to see more. My first two sales were to people who saw my work at Dad's reception. In an odd yet comforting way, I felt like he was still there taking care of me.

My new passion for chalk painting old furniture kept me sane over the next couple of months. I desperately needed something to grasp onto because everything else in my life was in shambles. Jenny and I were fighting. I was frustrated with my other two siblings because they wouldn't stand up to her. And Rob and I weren't getting along very well either. He was used to me being strong, and when I was down and hurting, my weakness upset him.

Two weeks after Dad died, we found out Mom was leaving Germany. She met a young man online, who was all of 21, and he convinced my 66-year-old mother to join him in Ghana, so they could be together. *That* was what Mom decided to do with the money she had coming now that she was receiving all of Dad's retirement. I was heartsick when I heard that, but I tried to just let it go.

In February 2016, I set aside my issues with Jenny, and we went to dinner to celebrate her 40th birthday. Two days later, I was getting dinner for my boys at Dairy Queen when she called again with the same line she used when she told me about Mom. "Are you sitting down?"

"What the hell's going on this time?" I said. "No, I won't sit down."

"I've been diagnosed with stage 2 breast cancer," she said.

Although we had been distant with each other for a while, this time we talked for at least 20 minutes. I reassured her I would do whatever I could to help her get through this. Later we found out the cancer had progressed to stage 3. Jenny fought her way through chemo, and as of this writing, she is in complete remission.

At some point, you'd think the difficult blows to our family would have to stop. But not too long after Jenny had survived cancer, the heartache continued. Aunt Marsha and I had again become close, especially after Dad died. The day Dad passed away, she called to ask if I was OK. As soon as I heard her voice, I broke down. Aunt Marsha showed up at my house with a car full of food and her infectious belly laugh. She prayed with us, and we shared fond stories about Dad.

We laughed recalling the time he went on a cruise with a few of his buddies. He was sharing a cabin with one of his friends, and they came in one night after having a little too much to drink and basically passed out dead drunk on the beds. When they woke the next morning the two were covered with a smeared brown mess. They thought they had soiled themselves in the night. But as they regained their senses, the men realized it was the chocolates the maid had left on their beds as part of the turn-down service. Laughing with my aunt really helped get me through a dark time.

Marsha began helping me with some of the chalk painting and furniture restoration. On November 3, 2016, I was supposed to go pick up some fabric from her house to restore a chair. She called to say that she wasn't feeling well and was going to lie down for a while. I could hear in her voice that she was tired and out of breath. I told her that I hoped she felt better, and that I loved her. She said she loved me, too. Three hours later, Aunt Marsha was gone. My cousin Mike called and said she died from a heart attack.

How could this be happening again? I was finally beginning to feel somewhat normal again for the first time since losing Dad, and then this hit. Another of my rocks had crumbled. Every time I started feeling a little better, another wave would crash over me, and I would feel like I was drowning all over again.

When I went to my aunt's house to be there to support my cousins, I was annoyed by how many people were there smiling and happy. I think that most of them were Marsha's friends and people from her church. This was just too much like when Dad died – there one day and suddenly gone from my world the next, and nobody seemed to care. My head told me that at least she didn't suffer through a prolonged illness, but my heart longed to say goodbye.

My cousins let me go into my aunt's room so I could be with her for a few minutes away from all the people. The coroner was there getting ready to put her onto the gurney. In the few minutes I had with my aunt, I knelt and through my tears said that I loved her and would miss her.

One of the paramedics was looking through her medications when he asked how long she had known that she was dying. He could tell from one of her prescriptions that she had to have known her condition was terminal. But she never said a word. Up to her dying day, Aunt Marsha wanted to take care of everyone around her but didn't want anyone to have to take care of her. This wasn't the first time I had wondered why Aunt Marsha couldn't have been my mother.

14

Mom's Got A Boyfriend

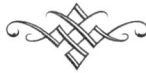

Three days later, while the boys were at school, and Rob was at his Dad's helping with a project, I was home alone staring at the walls lost in my thoughts. The TV provided white noise because I just couldn't sit there in silence. About 11 o'clock that morning, Jenny called, "Are you sitting down …?"

"What happened this time?" I asked, not knowing what dreadful shoe could possibly be remaining to drop on our family.

"Mom's been in a car accident in Ghana. They had to pull her out of the car. She's alive but not conscious."

"WHAT?" came my stunned response? "Is she going to be, OK?"

"They don't know if she's going to make it or not," Jenny said. "I don't know any more than that."

I didn't know what to do, but I had to do something. Even though I knew on an intellectual level that Mom had been dealing with mental illness for a long time, there was still a part of me that was angry and upset about how she had lived with us for so long and then left without saying a single goodbye to anyone. When I realized I might lose her for good, my rational mind understood my Mom had not been in control of her actions for all these years, and that helped me finally get over the heartache of a little girl whose mother had abandoned her.

I'm not proud that I had held onto that anger for so long, but this was the moment I started the forgiveness process that Dad had encouraged me to start years earlier. I began to understand the importance of unconditional acceptance of a loved one. I set all our emotional baggage aside because at this moment I just wanted to see her again, or at least do whatever I could to help save her life.

Although we hadn't spoken in a couple of years, I had an overwhelm-ing feeling Mom needed me to fight for her now more than ever. But what could a grocery store worker in California do for someone dying in a hospital in Ghana?

Desperate to find a way to help, I searched Facebook and somehow managed to get in touch with Mom's 21-year-old boyfriend, Nana. All I knew about him was that he met my mother on a dating website and had convinced her to move from Germany to Ghana to live with him. I learned quickly, however, that I couldn't always trust Nana. I may never know the whole truth about what happened to Mom the day of the crash. All I have is the story Nana told me.

"Your mother was depressed for a little while," he said in accented English. "She didn't want to leave the house." Which rang true with me because I had lived for years with Mom's moods. "I wanted to get her out of the house. I thought it would help her feel better. We had talked about coming to America to surprise your sister for Christmas, but I didn't have a passport. Your mother and I were driving into the city to fill out the application for my passport when the accident happened. We were going around a corner and one of the wheels of the car went up on a hill and caused the car to flip over. The car rolled several times. Your Mom was unconscious, and when emergency people got there, they had to pull her out of the car."

Even then, parts of Nana's story didn't add up, but I was too dazed by the trauma and didn't think to question his facts. For weeks after the crash, I rolled the details of Nana's story over countless times in my mind. Only then did the questions begin to flow out of me. Did others see the crash? Who was driving? Nana? Had he been hurt at all?

I told Nana to let the doctors know Mom had a stroke several years ago but had recovered fairly well. I asked him if there had been any scans done – X-ray, MRI, anything like that. That's when he wanted to send those types of pictures to me so I could take them to an American doctor for closer examination. He said the advice from an American doctor would help the doctor in Ghana. I told him that is not the way the medical system works in the United States, but I wanted to do whatever I could for my Mom.

After that, things became a blur. I spoke by phone with Nana a couple of times, and his story seemed to change every time we talked. At one point, he told me Mom had been walking around the Emergency Room. Then another time, he said she was still connected to tubes to help her breathe. These details didn't fit together, but I didn't want to say anything to offend Nana because I needed him there to talk to the doctors, relay information, and do whatever he could in Ghana. I felt utterly helpless and completely confused about Mom's condition. Nana seized upon the desperation of my situation, and it wasn't too long before he started asking for money.

A friend from work who is from Africa suggested that I call the U.S. Embassy in Accra. Because of the time difference, it was about 11 p.m. before I was able to reach somebody in the embassy. They said Nana had already reported to them that a U.S. citizen was involved in a serious car crash. That made me feel a little better because it appeared like he was trying to do the right thing.

Ultimately, my chat with the embassy proved to be incredibly disappointing for the most part. After being bounced back and forth to multiple people, eventually I spoke with Margaret Bula-Duane. While she was sympathetic to my situation and provided a lot of background information about how the medical system in Ghana worked, unfortunately her message was not what I wanted to hear. Since Mom had been in Ghana for more than a year, she had established residency, which meant the embassy was prohibited from doing more than if she were simply a tourist visiting the country. Mom would have to be treated like anyone else who resided in Ghana.

Margaret explained that hospitals there could turn patients out if they didn't have money to pay for their treatment. She further explained that the doctors and nurses don't actually supply medications for their patients in the hospital. Instead, they write prescriptions, and the patient must rely on family members or friends to go to a pharmacy and fill the prescription. That's the primary reason why I had to make sure to stay on good terms with Nana. With no one else to turn to, Mom would need him to get medicines and anything else she required.

Margaret's biggest concern regarding Mom was how she would pay for her medical treatment. She asked me if there was anyone who would be able to help her financially. My siblings and I were mostly living paycheck to paycheck, and Mom's only sister had died six days earlier. "There's nobody who can help out much from our end," I said.

Mom was continuing to get Dad's retirement, and although it was only $3,100 a month, that information seemed to make a big difference to Margaret. While the hospitals in Ghana had the right to wheel people out who couldn't pay, the cost of treatment was far less than we would have expected in the United States – and possibly even negotiable. Margaret assured me that as long as there was money coming in regularly, Mom would continue to receive care. Hearing that was such a relief. I felt like I could breathe again.

Margaret then began asking about Nana. I told her how they met online and the big difference in their ages. She was concerned that Nana might not be able to manage everything that was happening, and I agreed. But I had no one else I could turn to at that point, so Nana was my lifeline to Mom.

The next time I spoke with Nana, he asked for money to pay for tests and medicines. I told him in no uncertain terms that I couldn't help. I knew he had Mom's ATM card, and he needed to use her money to make sure she got her care.

When I spoke with Jenny about Nana, she finally came clean and admitted telling Nana not to inform me or anyone else in our family about Mom's real condition. Jenny said she didn't want to stress us out. I was furious and didn't want to speak to Jenny, but I continued working more information out of her before immediately calling Nana to get the truth about what was going on. Only then did I learn just how dire Mom's condition was. She had a severe head injury with suspected brain damage and multiple broken bones.

Jenny and Nana had lied to me, so I couldn't trust either of them. I didn't know who I could trust to give me honest answers, or who would have Mom's best interests at heart. I was as lost as I had ever been.

15

(Alfred)

A Stranger Among Us

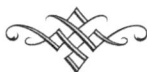

❦

I remember the day I met Katie's mother, Sandra Lee Pope, as clearly as if it was yesterday. I had heard about her presence well before I actually met her. Having an American patient admitted to our hospital – especially one in critical condition following a suspicious car crash – is not something that happens every day, so of course people were buzzing about having a foreigner in our midst.

Sandra was not initially my patient. She had not been placed in the Intensive Care Unit when she was first admitted, but I believe after a phone call came from the U.S. Embassy, she was moved to the ICU. That is how Sandra became my patient.

When I saw this older, white woman hooked up to a ventilator, I sensed right away that she did not have anyone here in Ghana to look out for her. My first thoughts were, "Where is her family? Who is caring for her? Who is responsible for her?" I knew that as Sandra's doctor I was responsible for doing whatever I could to protect her well-being.

When I asked around about who was with her, a hospital staff member pointed out a young man in the waiting room named Nana. Alarm bells sounded loudly in my head when I discovered the disturbing fact that Nana was Sandra's fiancé. It's not unusual in Ghana for some young men to prey upon naïve older women from other countries (*sakawa* in local parlance, i.e., online scams mainly targeting foreigners), so I did not trust Nana from the very beginning.

As I assessed the situation, a lot of things simply weren't adding up, starting with the fact that Nana had been in the same serious car crash that left Sandra in very critical condition clinging to life in a coma, while he appeared not to have any injuries. Moreover, why was such a young man from Ghana engaged to be married to a much older woman from the United States, I asked myself.

While I could not answer these questions with any degree of certainty, I felt deep down that Nana did not have Sandra's best interests at heart. I knew that I must keep an eye on him to make sure that he did not make any decisions that could further jeopardize Sandra's fragile condition.

That night I tried calling friends in the United States for guidance about what my next steps should be, but I was unable to reach anyone. I found the emergency number for American citizens to call their embassy in Ghana and reached someone there early the next morning. They already knew that Sandra was in our hospital but other than that they were not very helpful. I told them I was her doctor and would be willing to be the contact person for her family in Ghana because I sensed they should not trust Nana. They put me in contact with Sandra's daughter, Katie Stakolich, and that is how our journey began.

16

More Questions Than Answers

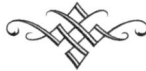

About a week after the crash, Mom was transferred from Trinity Hospital, where she had initially been taken, to Komfo Anokye Teaching Hospital in Kumasi. Margaret had been in touch with the new hospital and had made sure Mom would be admitted to the ICU by promising officials that Mom had the financial means to pay for her expenses.

When I found out that the physician overseeing Mom's case would be Dr. Alfred Aidoo, I immediately emailed him to establish some form of communication. In the email, I introduced myself to Dr. Aidoo and explained a little about our family situation. Alfred responded nearly right away with a phone call. He had a lot of questions about Mom and the circumstances that led her to be living in Africa. He wondered why an American woman of her age was alone in Ghana without any family members. I told him about Nana, and he was shocked by the age difference.

At this point, I did not know Alfred very well, but I sensed that I could trust him more than Nana. So, one of the next times we spoke, I asked him directly what he thought about Mom's fiancé at which point he admitted being uneasy about Nana's intentions. Nana had sent Jenny a picture of himself wearing a neck brace that he said was needed to treat the injuries he sustained in the crash. I sent Alfred a picture of the car after the crash, and he said Nana showed no physical signs of having been in a major car wreck. He continued that in the few days Nana had been hanging around the hospital he had never seen him wearing a brace.

I, too, was apprehensive about Nana's role in my mother's life even after Margaret assured me that in Ghana, they see couples with extreme age differences all the time. She said it was not really an issue where the embassy was concerned, and their relationship would not have any bearing on how government officials handled her case.

Having a doctor in Ghana who was familiar with what was going on agree with my feelings about Nana made me feel like I was not crazy. We both knew something was not right about Nana's story, but the justice system in Ghana works differently than in the United States. It is safe to say that we will probably never know the truth about the car accident and what really happened to Mom. Alfred did not think we could do anything about our suspicions without hard proof, and besides, our primary focus had to be on taking care of Mom.

Trustworthy or not, Nana was still useful in getting Mom's medicines and taking care of other errands. Otherwise, she had no one. Nana was aware of the fact that if Mom died, her payments from my Dad's retirement would stop, and the money train would stop. so it was in his best interest to keep doing his part to keep her alive. To further complicate matters, however, for some unknown reason Jenny was still putting her trust in Nana. This meant anything I told her would probably get back to him, so I had to be extremely cautious about what I might let slip.

While all of this was playing out in a hospital half a world away, I was also helping my cousins plan a memorial for my Aunt Marsha. Her funeral was beautiful but was also very emotional for me. I came home from the service with renewed determination to fight for my Mom. I stayed up all night thinking about Aunt Marsha, as well as Dad and Mom. I remember being awake so long that I saw the sun coming up the next morning. There was nothing that I could do for Dad and Marsha, but Mom was still alive, and I was determined to do everything I could to help her pull through. I may not have been the perfect daughter, and God knows she was far from the perfect mother, but she was my Mom, and nobody deserves to be alone in a situation like this.

During this time, I began to realize just what kind of unbelievably caring person Dr. Aidoo is. He kept me in the loop every day about Mom's condition. He promised to take care of her just like she was his own family. He even asked me to call him Alfred. He did all that he promised for my mother and for me. I soon discovered that Alfred is an amazing doctor and an even better person. I am so glad he was in our corner because I quickly understood that Nana was not to be trusted. Nana eventually started asking for money on almost a daily basis, supposedly to pay for new tests and medicines. I asked Alfred directly if these tests were really being done, and he told me that under no circumstances should I send money to Nana. In fact, Alfred said if Nana asked me for money again, I should forward the messages to him.

Nana was angry when I refused to send him money. He started insulting me and saying things like, "Your mother was right about you. You are a horrible person who does not care about her. If you love her, you would send the money." This sealed the deal. I decided right away to ignore Nana's abuse and rely on Alfred.

Over the next few weeks, Mom's condition did not improve as we had hoped, but I did make progress with the American Embassy. On more than one occasion, both Alfred and I had been hung up on by one person or another at the embassy. Alfred couldn't understand why they didn't do more to help. He had seen other medical cases where the officials at the embassy had been much more proactive. We eventually concluded that our lack of money and contacts of consequence definitely affected the officials' involvement in the case.

After I had been working with Margaret for about three weeks, she called at around 3 a.m. "Who is Jenny?" she asked. "She's my sister, why?" I said. "She called me, and said that she is Sandra Pope's oldest daughter, and I should be talking to her about Sandra's condition. I told her that I had been talking to you for the past three weeks. She hadn't been in contact before because she is dealing with stage 3 breast cancer. She says she is in charge of your mother's affairs. I can't report to both of you. I need to have one person to contact."

I could tell that Margaret was frustrated, and so was I. I thought by doing what I could for Mom, it helped let Jenny focus on her treatments. I feel a little guilty saying this because I know that she was dealing with cancer, but it annoyed me that as soon as Jenny could, she wanted to take control. This confusion made the process even harder. It felt like we were taking two steps backward in dealing with the embassy.

"What do you need me to do?" I asked Margaret. "There's some paperwork that you will need to fill out and have your siblings sign so I know who I should contact about your mother. Then you need to get it notarized and sent to our office in Virginia. E-mail a copy to me too, and then I can start communicating directly with you again."

Great, I thought, just what I need right now – one more thing to deal with. Why does my sister have a compulsive need to control everything? Not long after I got off the phone with Margaret, Alfred called. He was more upset than I had ever heard him. He almost sounded defeated. "Your sister Jenny called me. She wanted to talk about your mother's burial arrangements. I was angry with her. I told her that I deal with the living and your mother is very much still alive. If she wants to talk about her death, she could talk to Nana about that."

That was the first time Alfred considered walking away from helping my family. "Please don't give up on us," I said. He sensed how upset I was and how much I needed him. "I will still help your mother," he promised, "but only because of you and what you are doing for her." "Thank you," I told him sincerely, relieved that even if I couldn't speak with the embassy, I knew that I still had Alfred.

For the past three weeks, I hadn't slept through the night. I was beginning to feel like a zombie, and I was starting to crack. Mom's condition hadn't changed at all recently, and I was comforted knowing Alfred was watching over her. So, for the first time in quite a while, I turned my phone off completely and lay down next to my boys and got almost a full night of sleep.

The next morning, I got the boys off to school and then turned my phone back on. Immediately, the embassy called, and I saw that I had missed multiple calls from both them and Alfred. Mom had taken a turn for the worse and was bleeding out. A feeling of dread came over me, and I knew right away that she wouldn't get better.

I called my boss twenty minutes before my shift was supposed to start and told him I wasn't going to make it in. At first, he seemed annoyed. "The U.S. Embassy in Ghana called me and said my Mom may die today!" I snapped. "I need some time off right now."

His attitude changed quickly. "I'm sorry. Is there anyone you can talk to?" he asked. "Everyone I could talk to is dead," I said. I felt alone and empty inside. Rob never really liked my Mom, so he was no support. Why was this happening to me and my family? I felt like everyone was against me – family, my work, the embassy, and even me.

My boss listened compassionately as I poured my heart out to him. "I don't completely understand this myself, but I know that I'm the one who has to live with the consequences of every decision I make from this point on. My conscience won't let me just walk away and let my mother die alone." My boss knew a little about the situation with my mother's condition over the years, so it came as little surprise when he mentioned something about her karma. "I think she's definitely gotten her karma," I said. Still, despite all the history and bad blood between us, I still felt responsible for her in her final days.

I went to see my family doctor who had also been my Mom's doctor and knew of her mental health issues. I opened up and told her about what had been happening with my mother and me. It felt really good to talk to someone, even if it was only briefly. The doctor immediately signed off on my leave of absence from work. I started getting a little more regular sleep and began feeling slightly better. But I also knew it was only a matter of time now for Mom.

17

The Last Goodbye

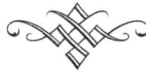

(Katie)

I was wide awake restoring a chandelier when Alfred called at 1:30 in the morning on the day Mom died. I knew right away when the phone rang in the middle of the night it could only mean one thing. "Katie, your mother's blood pressure is very low," he said. "It's hard to talk right now but stay by your phone. I will call you back soon."

About 20 minutes later, Alfred called again. "It's time to talk to your Mom now," he said gently. With tears streaming down my face, I poured my heart out to my dying mother. "I love you. I'm so sorry I couldn't get to you. I'm so proud of you. You're not alone. Alfred is there holding your hand for me. He loves all of us. It's OK for you to go now if you want to."

I didn't want to stop talking to her. I knew this would be the last time I would ever speak to my Mom when she could possibly hear me. At some point, I sensed she was gone, but I kept talking anyway. The words poured out of me in jumbles of emotion, but I couldn't stop. I probably told her that I loved her and that I was sorry at least 20 or 30 times. "You're going to Heaven now to see Aunt Marsha, Dad and your parents. I will see you soon. I promise. It's OK. I love you."

"Your mother passed away, Katie," I heard Alfred's soft voice on the phone again.

"Do you promise that she was there when I first got on the phone?" I asked.

"Yes, she was there, Katie," Alfred said. "I promise. She waited for you. I'm proud of you. I want to make sure that you'll be okay. I'm so sorry, but I have to go now."

"Thank you," I replied.

I immediately went into Rob's room where Mason had fallen asleep with his Dad. I woke Rob up sobbing and told him Mom had passed away. I really needed him to be there for me, but he just mumbled something and then rolled over and went back to sleep.

I was very upset with him at the time. I needed his shoulder to lean on while I dealt with my grief. Looking back, I really can't blame Rob for his lack of sympathy. Mom had not made it easy on any of us, especially Rob. She wasn't a positive influence in my life, and she certainly hadn't helped our marriage during the time she lived with us.

I went back into the family room and stared blank holes into the phone for what felt like a long time but was probably only a few minutes. I was emotionally drained and didn't want to talk to anyone.

I knew that I should call Stephanie back, but after Rob's callous response to the news of Mom's death, I was afraid others might react with similar indifference. I was on the edge of breaking down. For one of the few times in my life, I didn't know what to do.

When I looked up, there was Ryder standing beside me. Even without me saying a word, he could tell that something was wrong. "Mom, you look like you need a hug," he said, wrapping his arms around me and telling me that I was an amazing Mom. I was so proud of my son. He knew that I needed him and didn't ask any questions. A wonderful feeling of peace came over me. A few minutes earlier, I was almost ready to give up on everything, but I realized that I needed to keep going for Ryder and Mason. At that moment, I really did feel like God had sent me His tender mercy.

God has always given me signs when I needed them to keep going. He knew that without these signs, I would have broken long ago. My boys were signs, and Alfred was another. I have always had a vague belief in God, but Alfred's influence in my life has helped solidify my faith. I'm not sure what God's plan is for me, but as I hugged my son just minutes after Mom had slipped away, I really felt like my life had a sense of purpose.

(Alfred)

I cried the day Katie's mother passed away.

The other doctors and I were doing ward rounds that day when we noticed things were not looking good for Sandra. She was on ionotropic support receiving maximum doses of medication but still her blood pressure was dropping. She was getting close to a peri-arrest, so we would likely have to do CPR at some point.

I immediately sent a message to Katie telling her that the signs did not look good for her mother and to start preparing herself for the outcome. I called and then she called back. I set the phone down on the hospital bed by her mother's head and put it on speaker so Sandra could hear her daughter's voice for the last time. That's what I had done all the other times when Katie would call to check in with her mom. I'd put my phone on speaker and lay it by her mom's ear, so Katie could talk to her.

I drew the curtains snugly around the hospital bed forming a cocoon of privacy around Sandra so Katie could say her final goodbyes with the reverence they deserved. By this point, she was clearly barely hanging on to life. Katie kept saying that it was OK. Everything was fine. It was OK to go. These were very, very, very peaceful, loving words from a daughter to her mother.

This is precious. This is precious. Despite the distance and all the difficulties that her mother had imposed on her for most of her life, Katie had the courage and fortitude to offer grace to her mother as she was passing out of this life. It was good that the last voice Sandra would hear was her daughter and not the chaos of screaming physicians shouting names of drugs, while trying frantically to save her life in a sterile hospital room.

This was a remarkable thing that Katie did. The phone was loud and close to Sandra's ear, so I'm sure the last voice she heard on Earth was her daughter far away in California, telling her everything was OK, and to finally be at peace. This is precious.

Sandra's death was very emotional for me. Over a brief period of time, I had grown very close to her and her family. As their shepherd, I carried the weight of their sadness with me constantly throughout the ordeal. Right after Sandra died and I had made sure Katie was going to be OK, I went to the private doctor's room and wept great tears as I sat all alone with my sorrow. Yes, it was very sad.

I know in my heart of hearts, that even if only a few of the people who read these words are inspired to improve the lives of those around them, then Sandra Pope will not have died in vain.

18

Help Arrives Too Late

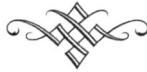

On the day Mom died, Margaret and a few other officials from the embassy were just hours away on a trip to check her welfare. It would have been the first time they saw her in person even though she had been in the hospital for more than five weeks. I can't blame Margaret for not coming sooner. Legally, the government considered Mom a resident of Ghana, so officially they were not supposed to make the trip at all.

Even though Nana had assured us he was taking care of all Mom's medical needs, neither Alfred nor I trusted that his motives were the best when it came to her. We told the embassy as much but because of Mom's residency status, officially their hands were tied. Consequently, the responsibility for questioning Nana about his intentions concerning my mother fell to Alfred and the hospital CEO. Nana swore to them he wanted to help her, but neither of the two interrogators were buying his story. They threatened to use their influence to "red flag" Nana's passport, if he didn't contact the embassy immediately and ask for help.

After that confrontation, Nana called me in tears with a full-on sob story about his meeting. I told him he had to do the right thing and call the embassy and speak to Margaret. Once again, Nana broke down on the phone while talking to Margaret. He admitted that he was young and as a result was in way over his head. He told her he needed help to care for my Mom, who was in fact an American citizen. That admission by Nana that Mom was an American gave Margaret the legal standing she needed to organize a welfare check for Mom.

Getting this admission might prove to be the easiest part of the mission. The four-hour trip from the embassy in Accra to Kumasi where Mom was in the hospital was not always safe for government officials to make. The funeral of the wife of one of the local tribal chieftains caused a short delay. Further complicating the matter was the 2016 Ghanaian presidential election that threw the country into a state of uncertainty when incumbent president, John Mahama, was ousted by Nana Akufo-Addo on December 9. Because of the political turmoil, government officials were not allowed to travel until things settled down.

After the election was complete and it appeared that there would be a peaceful transfer of power, Margaret was finally able to organize the overland journey to check on Mom in the hospital. She and three of her colleagues arrived just a few hours after she had died on December 13. Margaret called me around 4 a.m. I was still crying on and off and hadn't slept since getting off the phone with Alfred.

"I'm very sorry about your mother," she said. "I don't think there was anything we could have done, but I wish we had been able to get here earlier."

"It's OK, I know you are doing the best you can," I said. "I'm glad you're there now because I have no idea what to do next. What do I do now?"

"I can collect all your Mom's things for you. I will get her passport and any other paperwork that she has," she said.

"I think Nana has all Mom's things," I said. "Could you make sure to get her ATM card and her iPad from Nana, please? I'm sure that he's already taken all the money, but I don't want him to keep any of her things."

"Yes, I'll get everything I can," Margaret assured me. "I'll have to go to her house as well and even the site of the accident, but I think it's too late to learn anything there."

"Can you take pictures of where she lived for me?" I asked. "I want to see what her life was like."

"Of course," Margaret answered.

Nana gave Mom's passport, driver's license and ATM card to Margaret.

She identified Mom's body using the passport picture and description. "Nana's still in there holding your mother's hand," she told me.

"That makes me sick," I replied. I knew Nana was putting on a show for Margaret and the other people from the embassy. I also wished with all my heart that I was the one sitting next to my Mom holding her hand and not some scam artist.

After finishing at the hospital, Margaret's next task was to visit Nana at the house he had shared with my Mom in Techiman, about 75 miles north and slightly west of Kumasi. They found the house just outside of the town. Margaret later told me that many curious neighbors had come to see what was going on during the inspection. She said people, especially Nana and his mother, seemed nervous having them there.

"Katie," Margaret told me, "Where your mother was living is one of the worst places in this area that she could have lived. It isn't safe for an American. I can't believe your mother lived here for over a year. The house does have running water and electricity, but the electricity apparently goes out fairly often in this neighborhood. And there is no refrigerator in the house. She did have a bed, but she really had only minimal things in the house."

I wondered to myself if Nana had removed things from the house before Margaret had been able to inspect it. When Mom left my house two years earlier, I was as angry with her as I had ever been. I told Jenny that anything of Mom's that she didn't pick up right away, I would just throw away. Of course, now I regretted making that statement.

"Just please save anything you can," I said.

Margaret was able to get Mom's iPad, and I am grateful for that most of all. I have been able to go through the pictures, emails, texts and even some journal entries that she kept on the iPad, which helped me piece together at least a vague picture of Mom's life since she had left the United States.

This process of sifting through her belongings to discover her life made me sad, but I also needed to reconnect with Mom in some way so that I could have closure. After reading what she had written, it obvious to me that Mom was mentally ill. And, of course, I feel guilty that I hadn't been able to do more for her. I just hadn't been able to understand the scope of what was going on with her when she had been with me. Looking back over the breadth of her life, I now have a better perspective of how lonely she was and why she was always looking for a place where she felt like she truly belonged.

Margaret also gathered all of Mom's paperwork, some inexpensive jewelry, and shoes. She found a few dresses that were custom-made for Mom that Margaret said were costly. Mom had set aside one for Jenny and one for Angelina because she had planned to surprise them with a visit around Christmas. I specifically asked Margaret to look for the blue dress we had seen her wearing in an online profile picture. Ryder and I had both noticed how nice it looked on her, so we were pleased that Margaret found the dress and packed it along with everything else in a suitcase.

Next, she went to the store Mom had opened with Nana and his mother in Techiman. Margaret described the store as barely larger than a big closet filled with cheap merchandise that was worth a few thousand dollars. From the picture it appeared to be stuffed with inexpensive baby supplies such as clothes and walkers as well as a bunch of other items that you might find in a dollar store. From what Margaret could discern, Mom had originally paid for most of the merchandise, but now everything was in Nana's Mom's name, so we had no claim on any of it. Nana and his mother must have felt a little remorse because they gave Margaret a few items for Mom's first great-grandson, who was born five days after she died.

Before visiting the home and store with Nana and his Mom, I had the feeling that Margaret was giving them the benefit of the doubt. She was hoping that they were sincere in their intentions toward Mom and our family. But the visit completely took the blinders off of Margaret, and she saw them for what they really were – scammers.

While at the store, Margaret stepped outside so that she could speak with me in private. "Katie, I know you don't want to hear this, but Nana's mother says that your mother owed her $12,000, and she is asking you to pay off the debt."

I exploded and am ashamed to say that I swore for the first time while talking to Margaret. "My Mom paid for the lease and all the merchandise! I bet they've even taken all the money in her account and have left us with her medical bills! If she thinks she's going to get a fucking penny, she's crazy!"

By this time, Margaret was getting a little nervous about being in that location and wanted to make sure she left town as soon as she could. She visited the accident site, but as expected, after five weeks there was nothing left to see. To this day, I still have no idea where Mom's car ended up.

19

Mom's Money Is Missing

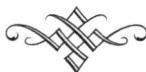

It turned out that Mom's possessions weighed 41 pounds and shipping them to the United States would have cost over $1,000. Margaret was kind enough to use her embassy account to ship everything so we could get a discount, but it still came to nearly $500. After getting the money together and sending it to Margaret for the shipping cost, it took almost three months for Mom's suitcase to arrive.

Jenny had enough of Mom's financial information so that within a couple of days she was able to contact the bank and she found out that Mom's account had a negative balance of $22 dollars. "There should be at least the $3,100 from Dad's retirement this month," Jenny told me. "Mom was in the hospital that whole time. What happened to the money?"

"Did you actually think there would be anything left?" I laughed. "Why do you think I've been fighting Nana the past five weeks? Of course, he drained the account."

As fate would have it, the day after we found out for sure that Nana had drained Mom's bank account, I received a call from him. "Katie, your mother had to be embalmed. The hospital already did it. It's a requirement for sanitation reasons. It cost about $200. Can you send the money?"

I could not believe his nerve. "What are you talking about? What did you tell the hospital?" I asked him.

"I said that your mother's insurance would pay for it," he said.

"No, you didn't," I shot back. "You know and the hospital knows that she doesn't have insurance. You told them to add it to the bill for her medical expenses – the bill that *you* have never paid, even though you are the only one who has access to her money."

"I don't know what you're talking about," he said, trying to sound innocent.

"Where is the money from my Mom's account? We talked to the bank, and we know there's nothing in there!" I was shouting by this point. "I know she should have had a deposit of over $3,000 on December 1st when she was in the hospital, and it's not there! Where is it?!"

"She had medical expenses," he started, but I cut him off. "You haven't paid any of her medical bills!" I said. "I've talked to the hospital and Alfred." Nana tried to stammer a response. "I'm done with you," I told him and hung up.

That was the last time I ever spoke with Nana.

20

A Salvation In Life And Death

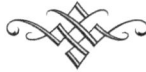

Margaret felt awful about the situation with Mom's finances, but there was nothing she could do since Mom had willingly moved to Ghana and become a resident. The hospital held firm to its policy of not releasing a body or even providing a death certificate until the patient's medical bills were paid in full, which meant Mom would have to be buried in a mass grave, unless through some miracle the situation changed. The prospect of leaving Mom in a mass grave forever surrounded by strangers was beyond unacceptable to me. It was bad enough that I had failed her so horribly in life, so I was adamantly determined not to fail her the same way in death. Her remains *would* be treated with respect.

For weeks Alfred had fought tirelessly to keep Mom alive in the hospital, and now he remained right by my side in an all-out effort to give her dignity in death. We had become close friends while Alfred oversaw her care in the hospital, but this labor of love to protect her in death had brought us even closer together. He had been my salvation when Mom was alive and remained steadfast to his commitment to our family during the time after her death, even when it wasn't clear what our next move should be.

"Katie, I don't know exactly what to do for your mother now," he said, "but we will figure it out together." I had no idea what to do either, but I believed in Alfred. His faith in God and my growing belief in a higher power allowed me to place absolute trust in Alfred.

I had planned to go to a friend's house to do some painting the next morning to get my mind off my worries, but while getting ready in the bathroom I was suddenly overwhelmed with emotion. I slid to the ground, crying and talking to my Mom. "I'm sorry," I sobbed. "I wish I could have been there. I wish it could have been different. I wish I could have loved you this much when you were in my life. I will fight for you, I promise. I will get you home."

At one point or another during her lifetime, everyone had abandoned Mom – even me. Things had become so difficult to deal with between us during the days when she lived in our house that I felt like I had to get away to protect my own sanity. But now that she was gone forever, I was experiencing tremendous guilt, so I decided my way of making amends for how terribly things had ended with her would be to somehow honor her in death.

During the days right after Mom died, I cried nearly every time I drove anywhere by myself. I was drowning in sadness, confusion and frustration because my world had become so hopeless. The car was my sanctuary. It was the one safe place where I could let go of my emotions and allow everything to flow out of me without worrying what others might think. Mom's death was the final blow in a series of rapid-fire gut punches I had endured in a very short time, starting with my mother-in-law's unexpected passing, then losing Dad and finally saying goodbye to my dearest aunt. I felt like none of my friends or family understood, or even cared about the terrible grief I was suffering with the loss of my Mom.

Our family started a GoFundMe page to help cover Mom's medical expenses and hopefully get her body back to us. Friends were generous, and we raised about $3,000, but we were far short of the more than $12,000 that we owed the hospital.

While Alfred and I started brainstorming ways to keep Mom from being buried in a mass grave, he suggested I write a letter to the CEO of the hospital, Dr. Joseph Akpaloo, asking for his help. I agreed to do it because Alfred thought it might help, but I'll admit the prospect of writing a letter to a total stranger left me paralyzed with fear. I've never been a good writer, and it scared me to death to even think about attempting to put all these swirling emotions down on paper. How could someone like me, a life-long grocery store worker with a high school education, even begin to tell Mom's story in a manner coherent enough to sway the decision of a hospital CEO so that he would grant our family mercy?

I was so afraid of writing this letter that I must admit I avoided Alfred for the first time in our friendship. For the next two weeks, whenever he messaged me, I either briefly responded or ignored his text. I didn't have the confidence to write the letter. I was so desperate, I seriously considered asking Jenny to write the letter, but something kept telling me her words wouldn't be able to convince the CEO. Deep down, I knew the letter had to come from me.

"You're not going to write the letter, are you?" Alfred texted me after I ghosted him for two weeks. His frank words killed me inside, but they also lit a fire under me. I had promised Mom I would do whatever I could to bring dignity to her death, but at the first sign of adversity I was hiding like a scared child. I can talk to people in person, no problem. Seeing their faces makes it easier to communicate. I sat down and tried writing, but the words would not come out. The cold stare of a blank sheet of paper made me speechless. "I can't do this," I thought to myself. "I don't know where to begin. I don't know how to make us sound like the kind of loving caring family that is worth helping."

"Just breathe. You can do this," Alfred told me. "Make it a timeline. Just pick a date and write about what happened on that day, and then continue from there."

So, I chose the day when Mom moved in with me and my family and wrote about that. When I finished with that, I picked another day. And then another. And I just kept going from there. While the letter writing process still wasn't easy by any means, ultimately the words slowly started to flow. It took me three days to put down on paper all the thoughts and emotions that needed I thought the CEO needed to know about our family situation.

In the end, the letter was close to three single-spaced pages long, and while I had successfully managed to put my thoughts down in writing, the message was a jumbled mess. When I read the letter it made no sense, which is bad since these were my words. When I asked Rob for help, he graciously counseled me on ways to clarify the message, so my thoughts were more cohesive and easier to understand.

I had no idea whether the CEO would even bother reading the letter, let alone care enough to help us. But since I had gone to the trouble of writing the letter and reliving all the pain of Mom's story, I was determined to make sure the letter made it into the CEO's hands. The only way I could think of to ensure delivery was to take the letter to FedEx. Sending a letter to Ghana with tracking cost me $130, but what else could we do? This was our last best hope. I knew the letter could make or break all our efforts to bring Mom home, so I prayed to God the CEO would get the letter and read it.

I handed the letter to FedEx, and then I waited.

21

A Surprise Gift From Ghana

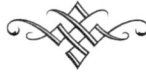

I was standing in my kitchen one morning about a week after I sent the letterwhen Alfred sent me a picture from Ghana. He was holding my letter to the CEO. The accompanying news wasn't just good, it was great. The CEO hadn't just gotten my message, he had agreed to help us bring Mom home. The news took my breath away, and I fell to my knees and thanked God. "We did it," I told myself, "This will change everything. Mom won't have to be buried in a mass grave after all."

I couldn't contain my joy, so I called Eddie and shared the great news. "How's he going to help?" Eddie asked, excitedly. "I don't know exactly, but I trust Alfred," I said.

In the end, I couldn't have been more thrilled with the offer the CEO made us to resolve the situation. Mom's medical bills were over $12,000 – an amount I'm sure would have been much higher had she been cared for in a hospital in the United States. Regardless of the cost, neither I nor my siblings had the means to pay the full $12,000 bill. Alfred and the CEO worked out a deal, and in the end, he agreed to settle Mom's bill for the $3,000 that we raised on the GoFundMe page. Finally, they could issue a death certificate and release her body.

Such generosity has rarely, if ever, been extended to an American family. I learned that in past dealings with Americans, hospital officials felt patronized, and the visitors were unappreciative and displayed a sense of entitlement. In my letter, I tried to be as sincere and humble as possible, thanking both Alfred and the hospital for everything they had done for my mother. When I asked the CEO if he would review Mom's file, I specifically told him how appreciative I would be for whatever he could do for us. I learned later that my gracious tone resonated with CEO and informed his decision.

Alfred knew the cost of sending Mom's remains home would still be very steep, so in an act of immeasurable kindness he asked a local tribal leader from Kumasi if she could be buried on their sacred land. At first the leader flatly resisted because such a thing simply was not done for foreigners. But Alfred explained how hard we had been working and told the man how close he and I had become. He explained my family did not have the means to send Mom's remains home, but we were hoping to find a way to bury her with respect.

Eventually, the leader agreed; Mom would have an honorable burial in Ghana. Alfred impressed on me what a rare honor it was for this man to allow my mother – an American – to be buried on his tribal land. I was immensely grateful for the leader's generosity and kindness and to Alfred for miraculously making this possible. In addition to being a doctor, Alfred is also an ordained minister, so he offered to officiate at Mom's funeral. Alfred's wife graciously helped with planning the service and picking out a simple headstone.

Things were finally falling into place, I thought, and then I spoke with Jenny. I was so excited that the hospital would accept the $3,000 that I didn't even consider that she might have other plans for the money. "No, that's not how I want to handle things," Jenny said when I informed her about what was about to happen. "I want Mom's body sent back to us."

I couldn't believe my ears. Jenny was flat out refusing to give me the money raised by friends and family to pay for Mom's medical expenses. I began yelling at her, and she hung up. When she picked up again, I told her, "DON'T YOU HANG UP ON ME! YOU HAVE NO IDEA HOW HARD ALFRED AND I HAVE WORKED TO MAKE THIS HAPPEN! NO AMERICAN FAMILY HAS EVER DONE THIS IN

GHANA! DO YOU UNDERSTAND THAT?"

Jenny dug in insisting that Mom's remains be sent home. Jenny and I fought over this for at least two days, and in the meantime Alfred had gone silent. It just wasn't like him not to respond to my messages. When I finally heard from him, he confided that the whole tumultuous situation with my family was taking a toll on him. It was consuming time at his work, and it was taking time away from his own family.

When I told him how Jenny was acting, he was simply beside himself and wanted to give up on us for the second time. "I just don't understand your family, and I don't know how you deal with them," he said. "I feel like it's us against the world, and nobody else seems to care." Perhaps if my family had seemed even remotely appreciative, Alfred would have been OK with investing the time and effort. He had done so much for us, and now Jenny refusing to give us the money was jeopardizing everything.

"I'll make sure that Jenny gives us the money," I said. "If I have to, I'll let everyone who donated money to the GoFundMe account know that Jenny is refusing to use their money to pay Mom's medical bills. I'll tell them about what great lengths we had gone to so the hospital would accept what money we *did* have to offer."

I decided not to publicly shame my sister. Instead, I posted a picture on Facebook of Alfred holding my letter along with the following message detailing the generous deal the hospital had graciously offered our family to settle the debt.

Two weeks ago, I decided to take a chance. I wrote a letter to the CEO of the hospital in Africa where our mother passed away. I wanted him to know my family's story. I put everything into this three-page letter that took me three days to finish. Then a week later Alfred messaged me and told me the CEO received my letter and said he wants to help my family. I could not ask for a better way.

To honor our mother. I don't even know how to begin to thank Dr. Joseph, the CEO of the hospital in Africa. We have lost so much in a short amount of time, but we have also gained so much more love in a place I never could have imagined, Africa!

One day I will go to Africa so I can hug and thank everyone who have made this happen. Joseph, Alfred, C and so many more. They have changed my life in avery wonderful way, and I will be forever grateful.

22

What To Do With Mom

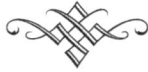

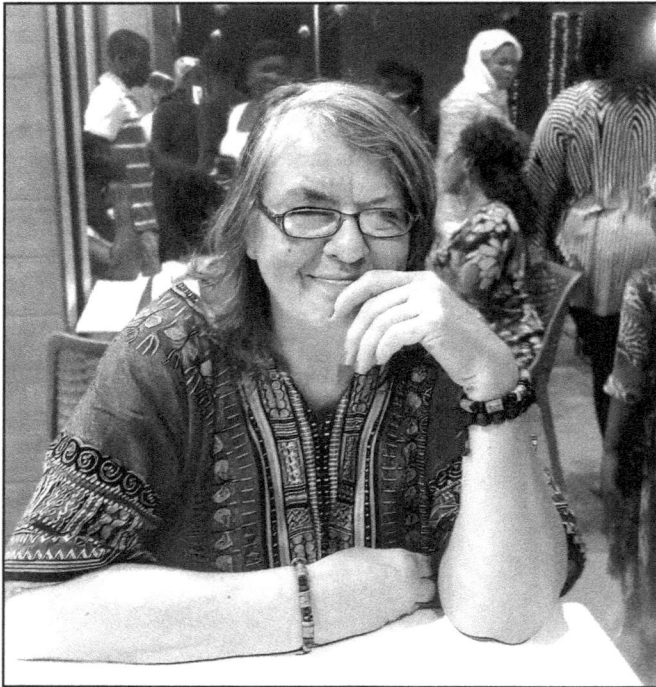

When a friend asked me on Facebook what was going on with the GoFundMe account, I explained that the money was going to be used to pay Mom's medical bills. Of course, this post made Jenny and Angelina livid. But I didn't care! I even fibbed a little to Jenny and said we had 24 hours to decide or lose the deal.

Everyone who wanted to have a say in the decision was invited to meet that night at Eddie's house. By seven o'clock, Eddie and I were there along with Jenny and Angelina, but Stephanie did not come. I think she just couldn't handle the drama of the situation and decided intentionally to stay away from all the stress. Once we all arrived, I called Alfred and put him on speakerphone.

"Thank you all for getting together so that I can talk to you," Alfred began. "I know that you all loved your mother, but I am disappointed that I did not hear from most of you while she was still alive. I have agreed to help because of what Katie has done both while your mother was still alive and since she passed away. We would not even be able to have this conversation if she had not written her letter to the CEO of the hospital.

To be completely honest with you, the fact that we even need to have this conversation at all, makes me doubtful and a little angry. If you do not take this generous deal that is being offered by the hospital, your mother will be buried in a mass grave, and there will be no death certificate issued.

So, you all need to figure this out right now. I have already used some of my own money and taken time away from my family in order to help you. However, I cannot continue to do this much longer."

"Thank you so much, Alfred. We appreciate all that you have done for Mom and our family," Jenny said, trying to make nice with Alfred, although frankly I knew he had run out of patience with her.

"You have to figure this out and give us an answer right away," he said.

After we had spoken to Alfred for about 45 minutes, he asked us to call the next day with our final answer. Once we got off the phone, we began discussing the situation and finally everyone agreed that we needed to pay the hospital the $3,000 using the money from the GoFundMe account. Even Jenny accepted the reality that if we didn't use the donated GoFundMe money, Mom would be buried in a mass grave, and none of us wanted that.

The biggest issue we couldn't agree on was what to do with Mom's body once it was released by the hospital. I wanted to accept Alfred's offer of having her buried in Ghana on tribal land, but Jenny had other ideas. She and her kids were adamant that we needed to have Mom's body cremated and her ashes sent home to California.

Historically cremation had not been an option in most of Ghana because tradition among some of the older tribal communities holds that burning human remains is not acceptable. But attitudes about cremation are changing, especially in larger cities where residents have adopted more modern views on the subject. Plus, as more and more cemeteries become overcrowded, cremation is becoming a more widely accepted option. This was definitely something we needed to consider, but we knew the cost might be prohibitive. The cremation and shipping would cost at least another $2,500, while the burial on tribal land in Ghana would have minimal expense.

"Where are we going to get the money to pay for the cremation and sending her ashes home?" I asked.

"I'll cover it," Jenny answered.

"*After* we pay the hospital what we owe them, right?" I insisted, speaking bluntly to drive my point home.

"Yes," she assured me. "If you have more money, don't you think we should offer it to the hospital to cover more of Mom's bills?" I asked.

Jenny didn't really answer the question, but she assured me that we would pay the hospital the $3,000 they had agreed on to settle Mom's bill. I didn't know where my sister planned to get more money. I still preferred to bury Mom in Ghana. Alfred had put in so much work to get the approval, and it was such an honor to have the tribal leader even consider this gesture of kindness. But at that moment, it just wasn't a battle I wanted to continue fighting, so I let Jenny have her way. The family meeting actually ended on a fairly peaceful note. I just wish I had known then where my sister had planned to get the money.

Jenny wired the hospital's money by Western Union to a bank in Ghana. Alfred had to take his 3-year-old daughter, who was sick, with him to the bank to pick up the money. But even this simple act of picking up money for Mom's hospital bills was laced with difficulty. Because of all the fraud cases and scams involving wire transfers in Western Africa, the bank wouldn't release the money to Alfred. I called Margaret to see if she could intervene. She contacted the bank, which agreed to release the funds if I could provide a letter signed by me authorizing Alfred to receive the money. In the letter, I had to specify the exact amount of money that he was picking up, but because the exchange rate kept fluctuating so frequently, I had to redo the letter multiple times. Finally, on the third time that Alfred returned to the bank with a sick toddler in tow, they released the money to him, and he was able to pay the hospital.

Margaret shipped Mom's belongings to me, and it took the suitcase over three months to arrive. I took the suitcase with all of Mom's possessions to Eddie's thinking it would be the easiest way to go through her belongings together as a family. I invited everyone to come over at the same time so each family member could choose something special for themselves to remember Mom by. Jenny never showed up, which didn't make a lot of sense at the time because she had made such a big deal about all of us going through Mom's possessions together.

It turns out Jenny went to Eddie's house later to look through Mom's things by herself. I didn't realize it right away, but she pocketed Mom's ATM card while she was there. I knew that after Mom died, Nana had emptied her bank account, so there shouldn't have been any cash left in there. But with all the delays in getting the body released and issuing a death certificate, nobody in our group had thought to tell the railroad company that Mom had died and to stop depositing Dad's pension money. So, the company just kept putting Dad's retirement money into the bank account for at least a month after Mom's death. As it turned out, the final deposit contained enough money for Jenny to cover the cost of cremating Mom's remains and shipping them back to the United States.

In order for Jenny to speak directly with Margaret regarding the logistics for the cremation and shipping, I had to give my permission. Frankly, I was so tired of fighting with Jenny by then that I granted my permission without giving the matter a second thought.

Even after all the things we had done, there was still one more hurdle to clear before Mom's body could be officially transferred to us by the hospital. When Alfred went to the hospital to make sure her body was released and loaded properly on a van intended to take her to a funeral home for cremation, an assistant to the pathologist met him behind the morgue. The man said he could not release the body because the doctor demanded to be paid the full $300 for his services. Alfred spoke on the phone with the doctor reminding him that the hospital CEO had agreed to the settlement and now the U.S. Embassy was expecting her body to be transferred to Accra for cremation.

Alfred had been so calm and collected as he helped me navigate through miles of red tape, but this time even he lost his cool as the doctor held fast to his demand for $300 before releasing the body. At that point, just to get this all finished, I offered to send the pathologist $300, but the CEO wouldn't hear of it. He told Alfred that I had kept my end of the bargain, and he didn't want me to spend any more of our money. The CEO, along with Alfred and the department head, all met with the doctor to make sure that he understood the magnitude of the situation. He finally agreed and signed off on releasing Mom's body.

Alfred sent me a video of him praying over Mom's body while it was loaded into the back of a hearse. I still cannot watch that video without crying. Alfred and I had worked relentlessly, and I knew in my heart that I had done everything in my power to provide a little bit of dignity to the end of my mother's mortal existence.

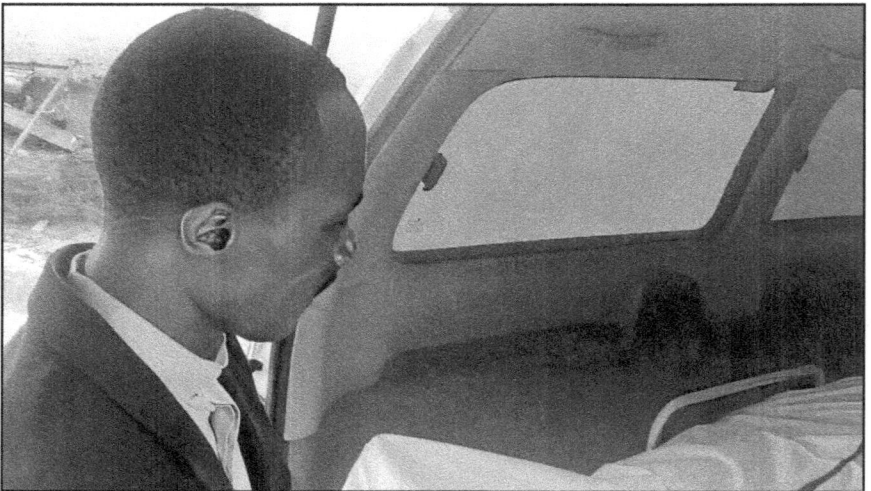

23

Jenny Takes All The Credit

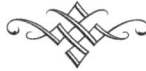

Almost six months later, we gathered in an upstairs room at The Old Spaghetti Factory to celebrate the high school graduation of Jenny's son, Shawn. There were about 40 people there – some of Shawn's friends, family members, but mostly Jenny's friends.

Once we all sat down, Jenny stood up to make an announcement. Of course, I was thinking she was going to say something nice about Shawn since this was a dinner to celebrate his graduation. Jenny's speech veered in a completely different direction that took me and everyone at the party completely by surprise. "I just want everyone to know that *I* went to San Francisco this morning. And *I* brought Mom home. *I* picked up her ashes from the airport!" she told everyone.

I could barely control my anger. I had specifically told Jenny in five different text messages that I wanted to go with her to San Francisco to pick up Mom's ashes. But she had ignored all my requests, and now she was taking all the credit as if no one else had lifted a finger to help get Mom's remains back from Ghana.

I stood up, hugged Jenny and tried to whisper to her quietly, "Why didn't you fucking call me?" I must not have done a very good job of whispering because everyone began staring at the two of us. I tried to rise above Jenny's pettiness and hurtfulness, but I couldn't stop the tears from streaming down my face. I went outside and began pacing in the parking lot. I called Alfred's number, but I couldn't reach him. I stayed outside until I felt like I had regained a little more control of my emotions, and then headed back inside. Halfway up the stairs, Jenny met me. "Aren't you so excited?" she asked, trying to make nice.

"Not only did you not call me to go with you, but you didn't even think of anyone but yourself," I snapped. "Didn't you think for a second that maybe this should have been a private family moment, so that we all could express our emotions without all of your friends staring at us?"

Several of Jenny's friends had shocked expressions on their faces after she stood up and quite unexpectedly announced at her son's graduation dinner party that she had been the one to ultimately bring her late mother's ashes home. She honestly believed that everybody was going to get on their feet and applaud her for what she had done. Quite the contrary, most of the guests appeared to be in disbelief that she chose this moment to make such an announcement. "You have no idea what your actions have done to Alfred and me," I continued. "Do you even realize what Alfred has done for us? He took time off of work. He had to take his sick daughter with him sometimes in order to help us.

"I helped him as much as possible from here, not you! You have no idea how much he sacrificed for our family and how many other people helped us because you weren't there and weren't a part of it!"

"I had to deal with the airport in San Francisco," Jenny began.

I couldn't help but answer in a mocking tone, "You had to deal with the airport? The American airport? That must have been *so hard* for you." Again, Jenny didn't seem to have anything to say, so I added, "After all that Alfred and I had done, I just wanted to be part of bringing Mom back home, and you took that from me. You have no idea what you just did, and even worse, you don't care."

When I went back into the party, it felt like everyone was staring at me, but the truth is they were probably looking away because I still had tears trickling down my face. I tried sitting down because my kids were still eating, but I just wanted them to finish so we could leave.

After a few minutes, I looked at my brother's wife, Mikey, and said,

"I can't do this." The two of us then went back outside. "I can't believe Jenny did this," I sobbed. "She has done so many selfish, uncaring things, but this is just too much!"

After a few minutes, I went back in to get my boys who had finished eating by then. "You're not going to stay for cake?" Jenny asked. "Nope, we're done," I replied. "I'm done, and we're leaving."

As I started to leave, many of Jenny's friends hugged me. They obviously realized how poorly she had handled the situation by excluding me from being part of finally getting Mom back home. At least somebody understood.

I knew Alfred would be upset when he found out about what Jenny had done, but the level of ire he displayed toward her surprised even me. "I had even been talking to her recently," he said, "and I had started to think that I had judged her harshly before and maybe she was a good person."

I knew that Alfred had been helping Jenny work through the details of getting Mom's ashes sent home. He had started rethinking his opinion of her. "I spoke with her recently, and she never said anything about going to pick up your mother's ashes," he said, appalled at her thoughtlessly callous actions.

"That's because she knew that you would have told me," I said. "And she wanted to take all of the credit." I knew seeing this type of premeditated selfish behavior was so foreign to Alfred because by nature he was never looking for credit or applause. Alfred had fought for us because he saw a family in need of help and it was the right thing to do, not for the attention or glory it might bring him.

"I don't say this to many people – because family is so important to me," Alfred said, "but you need to distance yourself from Jenny. She is so good at acting sweet, but there is always an ulterior motive with her."

24

(Alfred)
Changing Medicine in Ghana

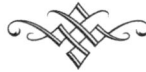

Thanks to the increased availability of modern medical treatments and an expansion in emergency care capabilities, we have made steady gains in treating diseases and injuries that previously would certainly have killed people at a younger age. Doctors are seeing an increased number of patients suffering from medical conditions more commonly associated with people in their middle and older ages.

The past decade has seen a shift in the kinds of major illnesses we see regularly in Ghana. While communicable diseases continue to be the leading causes of death, research shows mortality rates are on the rise for diseases such as hypertension, diabetes, cancer and stroke. Factors like urbanization, poor diets and globalization now come into play much more frequently than in the. So, on the plus side we're living longer, but on the downside, we're developing a whole new list of ailments.

In a country where a sizable portion of the population only has a primary school education, the burden of educating our citizenry about the importance of receiving regular health care falls heavily on a medical community that is already under extreme stress. To that end, I have periodically been the guest on a local radio program to help educate the community about health issues. We have also launched several programs to raise public awareness regarding health matters.

But despite our best efforts to educate the public, many still don't seek medical attention before it's too late for medical intervention to be effective. There are traditionalists who see the physical symptoms of an illness as the outward manifestation of a spiritual ailment afflicting the body. They generally turn first to various healers or pastors seeking a spiritual cure.

Unfortunately, when many of these individuals do show up at the hospital, it is too late for us to help. They have squandered precious time trying to find out what has gone amiss in their spiritual lives to cause their illness. We do our best to care for them, but when nothing further can be done, all we can do is comfort them and help alleviate their suffering. As a man of faith, I am perplexed. God has given us everything, including our knowledge of medicine. We need to embrace all that He has provided.

In Ghana, we have a major problem maintaining consistency and continuity among our leaders, which often adds to the mistrust and lack of understanding of the medical profession. We repeatedly experience shifts in policies and funding whenever the local or national political leadership changes. I have seen entire hospital projects abandoned after construction has begun due to funding being cut following a change in governmental leadership.

Every day, I encounter so many people needing aid or comfort that at times I become overwhelmed by the sheer magnitude of the despair in this world. In Ghana, we are very open with one another about our feelings and sharing life's burdens. It saddens me to the point of physical and emotional exhaustion when I stop to consider how little there truly is that I can do personally to ease the burdens of so many of my brothers and sisters.

God has given us all gifts with which we can serve others. As a doctor and a pastor, I try to give people hope that tomorrow will be a better day and the start of a brighter future. I treasure the times when I can help people find meaning in their lives because these are the most fulfilling moments of God's mission for me. When I started caring for Sandra Pope, I was trying to use my skills as a doctor to give my patient hope for a possible recovery. Eventually, however, I came to realize that Katie's need for emotional support and the lifting of her spirit was as great as that of her dying mother.

There are times when I question myself if the little bit of good, I am able to do is worth the overwhelming heartache and personal sacrifice. But then I meet someone like Katie, and I see what a substantial difference that my simple acts of kindness can make in another person's life, and my passion for serving others is reborn. Even though Katie and I were separated by an ocean, we were able to bridge the emotional and physical divide between us. We need more people who listen and care.

God has given us an arduous task to complete, and as a man of faith I will not shy away from the obligations. As the Apostle Paul once counseled the Philippians, I strive to regard other people as more important than myself. This is the life God has chosen for me. This is my responsibility.

A pastor who I greatly admire once told me, "A good shepherd must possess the smell of his sheep." What good is a shepherd if his flock is lost, and he is nowhere to be found? What good then am I as a doctor if when people are sick, I am nowhere around? As a shepherd, I hope that I will always care enough about my flock to carry the smell of my sheep.

As a physician practicing in an area of the world with limited resources, I must accept the challenges we face and do whatever I can to provide the best possible care for my patients. This does take a toll on me and my family, but I trust that God will bless us as we do our part to alleviate the pain and suffering of others.

Several times over the past decade, I have hosted exchange students at Komfo Anokye Teaching Hospital (KATH) in Kumasi where I work. In addition to my mentoring our visitors, we have also had the pleasure of introducing these students to Ghanaian culture. It was through these activities that I became friends with Dr. Mark Brouillette in 2010. We became so close, in fact, that I officiated at his wedding on my first trip to the United States.

Mark and I have been the leading voices in establishing a five-year collaboration between the University of Kansas Medical Center (KUMC) and KATH. We have helped coordinate and administer the Kovac International Observership Award, an annual all-expenses paid trip for one of the anesthesia doctors from KATH to visit KUMC to learn alongside their peers in a cutting-edge medical facility. Dr. Anthony Kovac Jr., a professor in the Department of Anesthesiology, Pain and Perioperative Medicine at KU Medical Center, who funds the award, has also donated much-needed equipment such as laryngoscopes, pulse oximeters and twitch monitors to KATH. He also bought thousands of dollars in medical mannequins to better train our doctors in intubation. He has come to Kumasi multiple times to teach courses in airways and anesthesia.

In 2016, Kovac told me about a new program of medical study in respiratory therapy that the doctors were establishing at Korle Bu Teaching Hospital in Accra. Most people do not realize the leading cause of death in Ghana is actually respiratory disease. But up until now, respiratory therapy did not really exist as a profession in my country. Of course, I knew about respiratory therapists and that they were very effective for providing in- patient care.

Kovac told me that after the respiratory therapy program was established in Accra, the hope was it would be extended to KATH. He suggested I go to Accra to see for myself what was going on, and that's where I met Lisa Trujillo and Karen Schell – the two women who, along with Dr. Audrey Forson, a pulmonologist at Korle Bu, have been instrumental in starting the country's first bachelor's degree program in respiratory therapy at the University of Ghana.

I immediately realized respiratory therapists could greatly benefit our patients, by providing new ideas and treatments. Plus, respiratory therapists are trained to treat common conditions such as asthma and COPD, which would reduce the workload of doctors and nurses who currently treat these conditions. The ratio of citizens to doctors here is estimated to be about 10,000 to 1, so any help we can get is much appreciated.

Trujillo was the Director of Clinical Education at Weber State University in Utah in 2005 when she met Albert Ncancer, a student from Ghana who was studying respiratory therapy. Ncancer knew her expertise as a registered respiratory therapist could provide much-needed training help, so he encouraged Trujillo to visit Ghana. She made her first trip in 2006 and immediately saw the need for respiratory therapy training in Ghana. She started Charity Beyond Borders, a nonprofit that organizes humanitarian trips for health care professionals to Ghana, and that's how she met Karen. As Lisa continued her trips to Ghana, Karen became one of her trusted colleagues, and eventually they both joined the faculty of the Department of Respiratory Care Education at KUMC.

By 2017, the first class of nine respiratory therapy students began the program at the University of Ghana in 2017. The students and some professors attended a month-long exchange program in November 2018 at KU Medical Center where they worked alongside their American peers, learning from experts in respiratory therapy. Eventually, this first cohort of respiratory therapists would graduate just in time to serve on the front lines of the COVID-19 pandemic as it swept through Ghana. I am pleased to report that as of this writing in 2022, the first batch is doing well. In fact, Joseph Boateng Makae worked so skillfully during his attachment at KATH ICU that eventually he was hired fulltime.

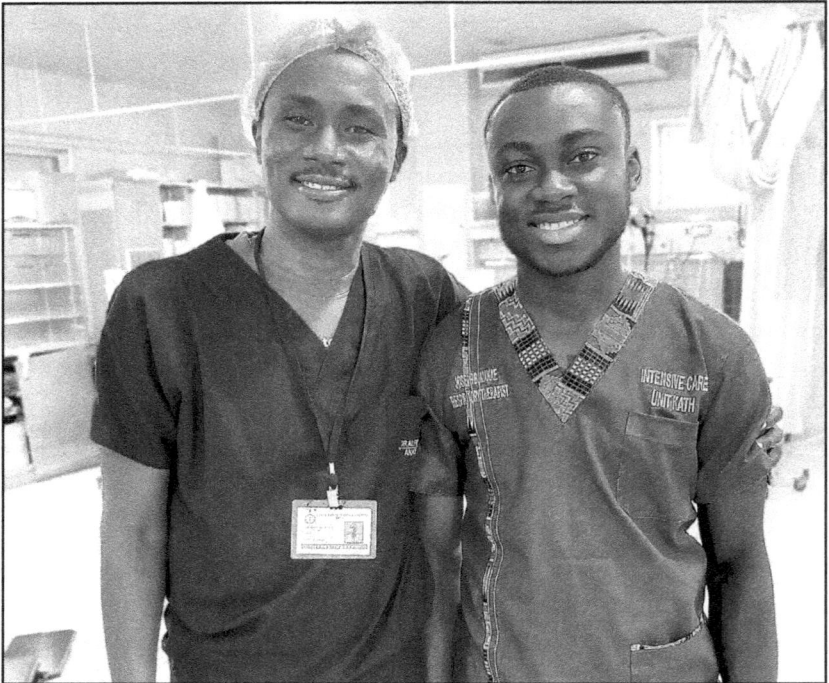

Alfred and Joseph Boateng Makae.

25

Cutting Through Red Tape

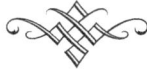

Apparently, during my visit to Accra, I had been so outwardly enthusiastic about all the promise that a new respiratory therapy program could bring to my country that Karen and Lisa strongly encouraged me to apply for an international fellowship from the American Association of Respiratory Care. Shortly thereafter I was awarded the fellowship. I was extremely happy to be chosen because the award would give me the opportunity and funding I needed to travel to the United States where I could see firsthand many of the more modern respiratory therapy techniques.

I would be visiting hospitals in Indiana, Kansas and Utah, but I have to admit, I also hoped that I would get to see some friends as well. Even though I knew that my trip would not take me all the way to California, I wanted to somehow get a chance to meet Katie, who had become my close friend even though we had never met.

The next step would be securing a visa – which I knew from experience would not be a painless process in my country. There is legitimate concern among officials that once people travel away from Ghana, they might not go back. As a result, the United States is very cautious about granting visas, especially long-term visas.

From Alfred's perspective, it seemed like the government was dragging its feet issuing visas. Here he was a doctor who wanted nothing more than to help people in his country, and he was having difficulty just getting permission to come here for training. He had tried unsuccessfully once before to get a five-year visa, so he was very familiar with how tedious the process can be.

I wanted to do anything I could to help my friend get his visa. I had learned a lot about international bureaucratic red tape while working on my mother's case with the U.S. Embassy in Ghana, so I called Margaret who had been extremely helpful dealing with our issues. I started by simply thanking her for all her support, but her response took me aback because it seemed almost apologetic. "I'm just sorry that it took so long to get your mother's remains home to you," she said.

"It's OK," I said. "I know you did everything you could. You and Dr. Aidoo were the only people who were on my side throughout the whole ordeal. In fact, I called because I wanted to talk to you about Dr. Aidoo." I told her some of the details that she didn't already know about how helpful Alfred had been to Mom and me. I also told her about Alfred's current situation and his frustrations obtaining a visa.

"What kind of visa is he hoping to get?" Margaret asked.

"He's hoping to get a five-year visa to travel to the United States," I said. "That's not easy to get," she answered.

"I've heard that, but he already has his fellowship in place, and he will need to travel to the United States for training multiple times," I said. "It would be so much easier if he doesn't have to apply for a visa every time he comes."

Finally, I told Margaret there was a part of me that felt like this might be my only chance to meet Alfred and thank him in person for changing my life so dramatically. I was on my break at work, so I knew I had to keep my composure, but as hard as I tried my voice cracked with emotion as I spoke on the phone. "I want to help Alfred. People need to know what he did for us."

"You should both be proud of what you were able to accomplish together," Margaret said. Tears of deep emotion began rolling down my face as I struggled further to hold myself together.

"Thank you," I said. "Can you think of anything I can do?"

"I'm not involved in the visa process, but you could try writing a letter to the embassy here in Accra describing what Alfred did for you and your mother," said Margaret (another person I would like to thank personally for her part in helping my mother).

I knew though that I didn't have enough time to write a letter and have it arrive at the embassy before Alfred's interview. But I liked the idea of writing something to help him. I have learned there is power in numbers, and Facebook had already helped me spread the story (I reached over 60,000 people in Ghana on Facebook using the boost feature to share his story), so I turned again to the power of social media in order to reach as many people as I could in a short amount of time.

Opening up my feelings to so many people is not something I'm very comfortable doing, but I knew that I needed to do it if I was going to help the person who had done so much for me. I decided to re-post Alfred's story one more time. I had sent the story out before, but most of the people it reached were from in and around Kumasi. So, I used what I knew about Facebook marketing to focus the target audience around Accra, the capital city where the U.S. Embassy is located. I knew I had to post something that people who were not familiar with the story could easily relate to.

Ultimately, I decided that the story was so important that I needed to share the details about the night my Mom died. I wanted the world to know about how Alfred had called me and then put me on a speaker using his own phone so I could say goodbye to Mom while he was holding her hand. These are my words:

*Hi, my name is Katie Stakolich, and this is
Dr. Alfred Aidoo. I want to share with you what he did for me
and my family.*

*On November 7, my Mom was in a serious car accident in
Ghana. Sadly, she passed away five weeks later from her injuries.
I know how much Alfred wanted to save my Mom. Some days it
seemed like he was with her for all twenty-four hours. The night*

my Mom passed away, Alfred called me and said I needed to talk to Mom. He put me on his speakerphone and held it up to her ear. I was able tell her how much we all loved her and how proud I was to call her my Mom. She was finally living life on her terms. I told her it was OK for her to go to heaven; we will be OK. She passed away listening to my voice and holding Alfred's hand. I wish every day that I could have been the one holding her hand. I couldn't have asked for a better person to be by my Mom's side in her last moments on this Earth.

This is just one of the many, many things he did for me and my family. This has been a very hard year for my family; we have had three deaths in 13 months —all unexpected and tragic. So, for Alfred Aidoo and the people of Ghana to help my family a world away is absolutely amazing.

It took almost six months for us to get our mother's ashes. This would never have happened without Alfred. I know how much time and hard work he put into making this happen. It was not easy with us being so far away.

My dear Alfred, thank you for your time, love, hope, so many tears, laughter and faith. How do you thank someone for this kind of love? I will get to Ghana to thank him and Dr. Joseph, who is the CEO of KATH teaching hospital. I know this would have turned out so different without the both of them. There can be so much bad in this world. There are also good and really, really great people. I am asking you to please share my story about these amazing doctors in Kumasi, Ghana.

Thank you, Katie Stakolich

26

'You Set Fire In Ghana!'

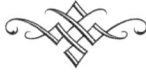

Right after posting the story, I went with my friend Rebecca and her family to a church retreat in an area that had spotty cellphone service. Before leaving, I prayed that God would help people see my post, and that it would help Alfred.

After we arrived at camp, I kept trying to check my post to see what was happening. Despite frustratingly poor cell service, I persisted and finally my dogged determination paid off. I was stunned when I saw we had reached almost 90,000 people and more than one hundred people shared the post. Among the hundreds of posted comments were numerous stories detailing how Alfred had helped their families make it through times of crisis. The majority of the comments were from Ghana.

"Wake up, Katie!" Alfred said excitedly when he finally reached me by phone the next morning at the camp. "Your post is trending here!"

He was right. In just over 24 hours my post had reached over 130,000 people. "WE ARE TRENDING!" I managed to say through my morning fog, perhaps louder than I intended. I wasn't exactly sure what trending meant, but I knew it was a good thing.

I nearly fell down in my haste to get through the zippered entrance of my tent as I rushed to share the good news with Rebecca. By the time I freed myself from the tangle of mesh netting that covered the door, I had tears running down my cheeks. Rebecca was also crying by the time I got to her. She had witnessed firsthand all my struggles with Mom and my family, so she knew how much this success meant to me. Still, we were both in awe of how fast the story was spreading to people around the world.

Later that evening, my phone was still going crazy with comments and notices about people sharing my post when Alfred texted. "YOU SET A FIRE IN GHANA!!" My post saturated the market in Ghana, but I didn't know how to deal with all this unexpected attention. I never imagined it would spread so far. The story was becoming bigger than all of us. The experience of my post being so well received made me realize with all of the negativity in the world, people needed to embrace some of the good things in life. I could see God's hand guiding us, especially as this ray of hope was emerging from something that had started out so tragic.

Alfred's words made me think about my life-long fear of fire, which began as a child when we narrowly escaped when our house was ablaze. When Alfred used the imagery of fire to describe our success, I'm sure he intended for it to be a positive thing. He didn't realize, however, that it might conjure up the boogie man of fear that has been hiding underneath the bed of my psyche since an early age. But this was different. This time, we had ignited a fire of the human spirit, and it was spreading a message of love to more and more people. This time fire was a good thing, I could feel my fear of fire melting away into the warm glow of personal accomplishment.

I had Alfred to thank for this personal breakthrough. Only by putting his well-being before my own was I able to stare down my inner demons of self-doubt and share so many intimate details about my life with such a large audience. We *had* set fire in Ghana – and this time the warmth of the blaze felt good.

God's plan for our lives isn't always clear to us in the moment when things are happening. But on this occasion, I'd like to think that He showed me the way to spark a blaze that could change the world – even if it's just a little corner of humanity. Eventually, my post would reach over 300,000 people. I know from the posted comments the fire spread throughout Africa, the United Kingdom and Norway.

On the last morning at the retreat, I attended a testimony meeting where anybody who felt divinely inspired was encouraged to share their epiphanies. Rebecca kept telling me I needed to share my story with the others, but once again I was terrified by the prospect of speaking in front of strangers, so I texted Alfred. "I'm standing there next to you," he messaged, while his words from the day before echoed in my mind. *"You,* started a fire in Ghana!" Suddenly, I felt the courage stir inside me to do what needed to be done.

If this fire were to continue to grow, I knew there would be more times when I had to leave my comfort zone. With Rebecca by my side and Alfred in my heart, I stood up in front of all those people and told my story about losing Mom but finding a blessing in Alfred. My hands trembled as I read my Facebook post and shared my excitement about how many people had responded. I shared how Alfred was trying to get his visa so he could help bring the respiratory care program to hospitals in Ghana.

In the end, it felt amazing to be able to talk about this in front of so many people. I was filled with a power beyond my own. I could feel God pushing me to stand up and share my story. Many people came up to me afterward and thanked me for my testimony and promised to pray for Alfred. This experience made me confront fears that I have been carrying around with me for most of my life. Fear of fire being one that I have possessed the longest. Since that day at the retreat, however, I have never had another nightmare about fires.

27

A Chance To Meet Alfred

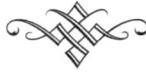

On July 31, 2017, Alfred made the more than four-hour journey to Accra to try once again to obtain a visa. As he went in for the interview, he sent me a picture of himself at the embassy. I could tell he was nervous, so I messaged him, "I'm standing there next to you."

Alfred had been through a visa interview before, and he couldn't believe how short this one was. The person doing the interview knew who he was and even seemed to already know some of his background story. Alfred was asked to state his name, where he was going, a quick explanation of the purpose of his trip, and when he would be coming back. That was it. Those were all the questions.

A couple of days later, Alfred messaged saying they gave him a five-year visa. When I saw that message, I cried tears of joy, and a sense of triumph filled my heart because this would help him in so many ways. This was huge for Alfred and his family. We were only expecting the embassy to give him a regular visa because the government grants so few five-year visas.

With Alfred coming to the United States, I knew there was a chance, however remote, we might meet face to face. I remember sitting on my bed feeling overwhelmed with gratitude and then the angst of uncertainty about how we could get together during his trip. I knew one of the places he would go on his trip would be the University of

Kansas Medical Center in Kansas City, Kansas. My friend Lisa lives about a half an hour away from there, so I quickly left her a message and then got ready for work. After my shift, I started planning my trip in earnest.

Alfred was still shocked by how easily he had been given his visa. He was also surprised by the local celebrity status he was starting to have after my social media post reached over 300,000 people, was shared over six hundred times, and received more than seven hundred comments. I felt a little guilty because I knew he did not really want so much attention, but he realized that this was a rare window of notoriety he could use to promote his efforts to help others.

Alfred's friend, Karen Schell, was one of those who saw my Facebook post, and she asked Alfred for more details about how we knew each other. He told her our story and then helped Karen contact me. We hit it off right away.

"I have an idea," Karen said after we had gotten to know each other better. "Does Alfred know for sure that you are coming to meet him in Kansas City?"

"I don't think he knows exactly when we will see each other," I said. "I know he's going to be pretty busy with all of his medical commitments when he comes, so I just want to meet him and spend whatever time he has to spare. I think he's visiting hospitals in New York and Indiana before coming to Kansas City, and maybe one in Utah afterward. I don't want to get in the way of the main purpose of his trip."

"Why don't we do this?" Karen said. "I have an apartment right across the street from the University of Kansas Medical Center. You could stay with me, and then you would be nearby to see Alfred whenever he has some free time."

"If you're sure that would be alright," I said. "I have a friend in the area, but she lives about a half an hour away. If I stay at your place, I could still see my friend, but I would be closer so I could see Alfred easier around his schedule."

"Then it's settled," Karen said. "You'll stay with me. I even have an idea about how you can meet Alfred."

I wasn't quite sure what Karen meant, but she seemed to have something in mind. "I was thinking that we should try to surprise him," she began. "Your story is amazing, and your post really touched me. I think other people should hear about this too. Would you be OK if I set something up at the university and maybe have a couple of reporters there?"

This idea simultaneously thrilled and scared the shit out of me. I hate speaking in front of people, so just the thought of talking to reporters and being interviewed made me feel weak in the knees. I even tried using Alfred as an excuse, claiming he wouldn't like that much attention.

"I know that" Karen said, "but just think about how much good it will do the respiratory therapy program to get some press coverage. We are all trying to improve medical conditions in Ghana and make some major changes. We need as much of an audience to help support this cause as we can get. The power of your Facebook post shows just how influential your story can be. Your story can help so many people in Ghana."

I knew she was right. I had to do whatever I could to support Alfred, the hospital that had been so generous to our family, and most important, the people of Ghana. "Ok, let's do this. Make the plans and let me know what you want me to do."

Karen called me once she had made the arrangements. "I'm sure Alfred is hoping to see you when he is here, but we'll have him think that you're getting here toward the end of his time in Kansas City. That way when he sees you for the first time, it will be a complete surprise."

I was so excited to meet Alfred, but I was also terrified about being interviewed. I also knew I would also have a challenging time keeping Karen's plan to myself for six weeks because I talked to Alfred almost every day.

The next few weeks felt unsettled. As the time drew closer for me to go to Kansas City, there were moments I honestly considered not going. It may sound silly, but I am a grown woman who had never travelled this far from home on my own. I had spoken to Karen and Alfred on the phone and online, but I had never met them, so this adventure was way, way outside of my comfort zone.

I remember thinking that the person I had been just a year earlier would have never done something like this but dealing with all the fallout from my mother's death in Ghana had reshaped a part of me. The situation with Mom had opened the door for me to have this experience, and while the two of us had many differences, she was never one to shy away from trying something new. In some strange way she had delivered me to this point. I had also begun feeling the presence of God more in my life, and that gave me comfort as well.

I had to go, and I knew it. If for no other reason than to be there for Alfred. I do not have the knowledge or skills to make the societal changes that Alfred can, but I needed to contribute something, anything I could to the goal of bringing respiratory therapy and improved medical care to the people of Ghana. So, if that meant facing my fears and giving an interview or two to further this worthy cause, I would do that.

28

Kansas City, Here I Come

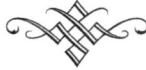

I boarded an airplane in Sacramento on September 19, 2017, and landed in Kansas City just after 10 p.m. Karen picked me up at the airport. We hit it off right away and visited just like old friends all the way back to her apartment. By the time I settled in and we finished talking, it was almost 2 a.m. "We have an early morning," Karen said. "You are meeting with a reporter from the university at 8:30 tomorrow morning."

After a day of traveling and a two-hour time change, I slept through my alarm. Karen finally woke me, and I rushed to get ready. We made it to the university on time, and the fear of being late left me no time to be nervous. "This is Greg Peters from University Communications," Karen said.

"'Wow, this is really happening,'" a little voice inside my head chided. "I don't really know where to start," I admitted.

"Why don't you just tell me your story – start from the beginning. I've got time," he said. So that's what I did. I told him the whole story about my Mom and her accident. I told him how Alfred had been there to help me through the whole thing. I told him how we had become such good friends even though we had never met in person. Finally, I told him about Alfred's desire to come to the United States and learn medical techniques, including respiratory therapy, which will help improve health care in Ghana, and I had done what I could to help him get here.

Of course, I used most of a box of tissues, but I got through it. The reporter listened almost without speaking. "I can't believe you two have done all of that together," he said. "And you've never even met?"

"No, today will be the first time," I answered. I noticed at that point that both Karen and Greg had tears in their eyes. "People need to hear this story," he told me.

After the interview, Karen showed me around the campus, and then we met up with my friend. Lisa. It meant so much that she was there. I was excited to be meeting new people, but it was also nice to have someone who actually had known my Mom and family. Alfred was scheduled to arrive at about 4 p.m. from New York, so Lisa and I went back to Karen's apartment to change clothes and get ready.

I was getting increasingly nervous and excited at the same time. It just did not feel real. I'm a little embarrassed to admit that Lisa ended up giving me two glasses of wine to help calm me down. Karen had told us where we needed to be in order to surprise Alfred, but on the way there, we got a little lost trying to navigate our way around the university. Fortunately, some students directed us to the building where we would eventually meet Alfred.

The area was very sleek and modern – not at all like I had pictured. There were maybe 20 people gathered on the Health Education Building Bridge, including Karen and the University Communications person I had met earlier. I was also introduced to a cameraman from a local TV station and a reporter from the Kansas City Star. We still had a little while before Alfred would arrive, so the cameraman began filming and asked me what it means to me to finally meet Alfred.

I honestly don't know exactly what I said or if it even made any sense. I do know that this simple question opened a floodgate of jumbled thoughts and emotions in my head. What did it mean to me to finally meet Alfred? Such a simple, yet tricky question. I could answer that in one of two ways.

The one-word answer is "everything." Meeting Alfred means everything to me! The longer answer brought a flood of memories and thoughts to my mind. Meeting Alfred would bring closure to the rocky, heart wrenching, life-defining relationship I had shared with my mother. Despite our relationship being so negative for much of my life, Alfred's influence tempered my recollection of Mom, so my memories were a mix of tender and bittersweet.

Plus, meeting Alfred now would hopefully allow me to play a small part in the work that he does daily helping people in Ghana. I thought about all the people who have reached out to us since they learned of what Alfred had done to help my mother and me. I thought about how I would be connected in some small way to the good Alfred accomplishes.

I thought about how our friendship may have changed this simple man as well. I had become somewhat protective of Alfred although I had never met him. He had become a local celebrity although he had never sought accolades. While Alfred shied from the limelight, he understood the more people knew about his work, the more good he could do.

The most important thing about meeting and getting to know Alfred was that the experience we shared had brought me closer than ever to God. Alfred and his faith guided my path. God puts people in our lives as answers to prayers and as blessings – Alfred has been both to me. Meeting Alfred that day would be the culmination of all the hours, tears and hope that we had both put into helping each other. In a sense, the two of us finally meeting felt like a tender mercy from God that made all the heartache and pain of the past year somehow bearable.

29

We Meet At Long Last

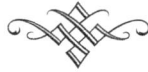

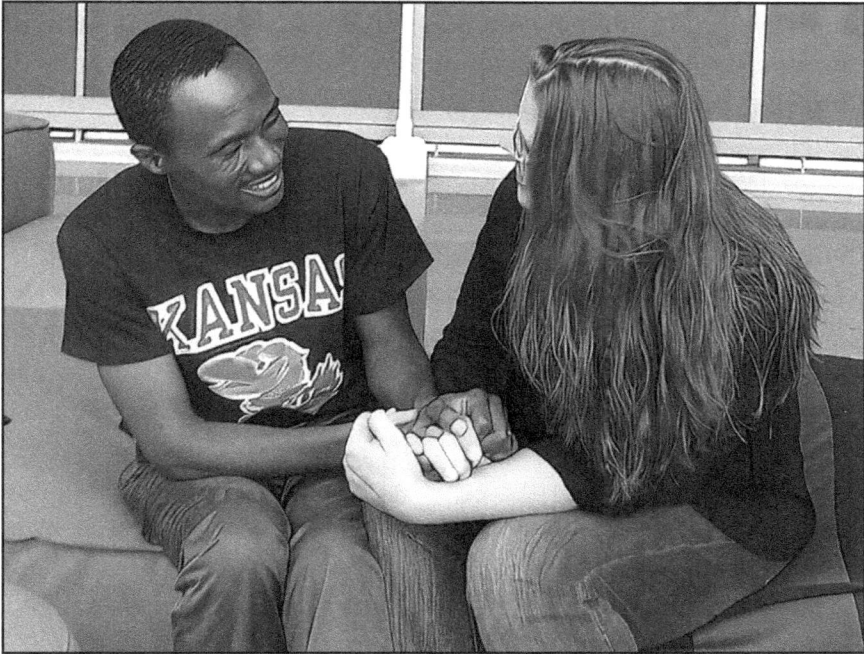

When the time had finally come to meet Alfred, I first heard his voice speaking to Karen as they approached where I was hiding. I was still extremely nervous and excited as I stepped out from behind a room divider and into Alfred's path. All of the sudden, there *he* was standing in front of me. My unexpected appearance from out of nowhere totally caught Alfred by surprise. He looked, with the puzzled glaze of a man who couldn't trust what his eyes were seeing. Then he looked again. "Katie? Is it really you?"

"Yes, surprise! It's really me," I said.

We stood there staring at each other for what seemed like an eternity; both of us caught up in the magnitude of the moment and neither of us daring to speak on the chance it might break the spell and awaken us from this glorious dream. Finally, I stepped forward and touched Alfred's hand. What a distance we had come after fate brought our worlds together – the doctor from Africa and the grocery store worker from California.

We hugged with the embrace of two people who had survived having the weight of the world on their shoulders for a long arduous journey that only they could comprehend. "We did it," I whispered to my old friend, who I had just met. "People will know what you did for my family – for my Mom." I put my hands on either side of his face and looked deeply into his eyes. "People will know what you have done."

Both Lisa and Karen had tears streaming down their faces, just like I did. It felt like I was watching someone else's crazy life unfolding on an episode of Dateline, I thought. I like watching shows like Dateline because they remind me that my life isn't the only crazy one in the world.

I had so much to say to Alfred, but it was awkward since we were surrounded by doctors, reporters and others who all wanted to meet and talk to us. At some point, the reporters began asking Alfred about my mother's story and what brought him and me together. "This kind of thing should never happen," Alfred told a reporter. "A family shouldn't have to go through something like this without more help. If nothing else, I hope any attention from this situation will help bring about changes that will help families in similar circumstances in the future." That was just like Alfred, already looking ahead at how what we had gone through could benefit someone else.

"How can this help humanity?" a reporter asked. The question stuck in my mind because at first

I thought it was so strange. I have no idea how this can help humanity.

After all, I'm just a cashier at a grocery store, I thought. God's power and mercy gave me words that I would not have spoken on my own.

"Hope," I said. "This gives people hope that there is good in the world. There are people who still care for others in the middle of so much evil and negativity. Open your eyes and see this hope. Let these people in. Don't block them out because of where they come from, the color of their skin, their background, culture or religion. We're all searching for hope. Doctor Aidoo gave me hope when I needed it, and just maybe our story can give hope to other people as well."

The same reporter asked another question but for an entirely different reason. "In your Facebook post, you mention that you had lost a few people close to you over the past year. Would you care to elaborate?"

That kind of knocked the wind out of me for a second, but it was a fair question. Talking about it might be a way to help others, so I fought to control my tears. When I looked at Alfred he nodded as if to say, "You can do this."

"I lost my Dad first, about a year ago," I began. "He was an amazing man, and I miss him every day. Then just as I was starting to learn to live with the pain of his loss, my aunt, who I was very close to, also passed away. Three days after my aunt died, I got the phone call about my Mom's accident.

"It's been a rough year, but I know that they are proud of me. I had to push forward to fight for my Mom. Alfred and God were there to help me to keep going. Sometimes, I felt anger and sadness, and in a strange way, these emotions pushed me as well."

Eventually, when all the questions had been asked and the pictures taken, I could finally relax. "Did I do OK?" I asked Karen. "You did wonderful," she said. Her words made me feel better because I worried that I had been a blubbering idiot. After everything slowed down, I sat on a couch next to Alfred with Karen. I reached over to touch Alfred's hand, wanting to make sure one more time that all of this was real. We talked for a little while, and it was amazing. But what I really wanted was to talk to Alfred without so many people around.

Alfred had just gotten in from New York, so he needed to eat something. He loves pho soup, so we found a Vietnamese restaurant and even I tried it for the first time. I know that may not sound like a big deal to most people, but this trip was such an opportunity for me to be away from my comfort zone and try new things. When our group arrived at the restaurant, we Face Timed Alfred's wife. She had no idea that all of this was happening and was genuinely happy with how well everything worked out.

"How long had you planned this surprise?" Alfred asked. "Six weeks," I said. "And it was so hard for me to not say anything. We talk almost every day."

After dinner, I spent time with Alfred and Karen at her apartment. We looked at Alfred's schedule for the following day to see when we could get together. He was pretty booked up with classes and lectures. "You do what you need to do," I told Alfred and Karen. "I will squeeze into your schedule whenever works for you." I was just so happy to have some time to spend with Alfred.

The next morning, I learned that *The Kansas City Star* had published its story about Alfred and me. I thought that the article would be more about Alfred and his efforts to build a respiratory program, but it turns out that my unusual friendship with Alfred and what we had done together for my Mom was the crux of the story. I felt silly, but I began sobbing as I read the story. I called Alfred right away, and he had seen the article too.

"Beautiful," he said softly.

30

Alfred Touches My Heart

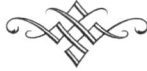

I was pretty excited the day Alfred gave his lecture to Karen's respiratory therapy students. Karen had arranged a lunch buffet where Alfred and I could meet some of the doctors and students. As someone who works in a grocery store, I was a little intimidated by this group, but everyone was gracious and welcoming.

"In Africa, we don't have all of the machines and tests that you have here, so we have to use our intuition more, and I think sometimes this is a good thing," Alfred began his lecture.

"You cannot always depend on technology to diagnose a patient. Machines can be useful, and they have their place, of course, but I think that as a medical professional, you become more observant and can better develop your own sense of what a problem might be if you do not always rely on tests and technology. However, whenever possible, you should use the technology available to confirm or even contradict what your instincts tell you is happening with your patient.

Alfred really touched my heart when I heard him speak in person about what he had done for me. "Something that often gets overlooked is the family of the patient. If they have a loved one who is sick or injured, the family will be stressed and worried as well. We can make sure that the family does not feel like they are going through this alone. There are many ways we can show them that we care and are there to support them," he looked straight at me and told the students.

Once again, I found myself being a little protective of Alfred. Having never attended college myself, I was expecting it to be more formal than high school. I did not imagine anyone talking or not focusing during Alfred's lecture, but a couple of young women within earshot of where I was sitting kept whispering to each other throughout the lecture. I was indignant on Alfred's behalf. He had come all this way to talk to these students, the least they could do was to be courteous and not talk while he was lecturing.

Alfred pretty much had the attention of all the other students, so he either didn't notice the women or chose to ignore them. On the other hand, I wanted to get up and say something to the rude women about their discourteous behavior, but I held my tongue knowing that as a guest it wasn't my place to call them out, so I just let it go.

After the lecture, several of the students wanted a picture with Alfred. One girl had noticed that he had looked my way a few times during his lecture, so she asked how I was connected with him. I was able to share a little of our story, and I told her to look for the article in the newspaper if she wanted more details. That was a pretty cool feeling.

Alfred had such a busy schedule, and I knew that he was tired, so I decided to let him get some much-needed rest, while I went out with Lisa and her friends to the Belvoir Winery. It was good to relax and converse with the others. I told them stories about the people I had lost and how Alfred had been there for me during Mom's ordeal. I could tell they were touched by my words, and several of them shared memories of loved ones they had lost.

I spent the night at Lisa's house, and that was great because I was able to sleep in and visit a little with her. Alfred was busy in meetings and training all day, so we were in no hurry. Lisa drove me back to Karen's, and that gave me a chance to do some grocery shopping before Karen and Alfred finished their day.

I wanted to do something special for Alfred and also to thank Karen for letting me stay at her apartment, so I had offered to make dinner at Karen's that evening. I made a taco bar for Alfred, Karen and some of her family who had joined us. Alfred commented at one point that evening, "I cannot believe that I am actually here with two of my favorite people in the world, and Katie is cooking me dinner. I am a lucky person."

After dinner, we sat in the small living room and soon I could feel everyone's eyes fixed on Alfred and me. I looked at Alfred and asked if it was time to tell them our story. "Yes!" they all shouted at once. Karen and her family hung on our every word as we told our story together for the first time. At one point, I looked up and all of them were crying. I believe our story is powerful when either of us shares it by ourselves, but the feeling is magnified and more complete when we tell it together.

The trip made me realize I actually enjoy being pushed outside of my comfort zone and experiencing new things. So that evening I made a pledge, I would no longer let my feeling uncomfortable or a little nervous stand in my way of doing the things I needed to do. This book is evidence of that.

31

Just The Beginning!

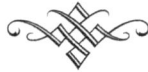

The next day, we took Alfred to a Renaissance Festival. He was excited to see the jousting despite the oppressively hot, humid Kansas weather. I am in awe of his boundless energy and enthusiasm. In some ways, he reminds me of an innocent child who is full of wonder about the world around him. He was totally fascinated by all the costumes that ranged from historically authentic to more of a fantasy version of a true Renaissance outfit. Alfred was both amused and bewildered why Americans would celebrate such a somewhat skewed and idealized version of European history.

Karen and I wanted to buy matching dresses and headbands for Alfred's daughters, but he didn't want us to spend our money on him or his family. We finally had to kick Alfred out of the shop, and then we bought the dresses. We had an amazing day together.

That evening, I attended a barbeque with Karen and Alfred at the home of one of the doctors from the hospital. He was a very friendly man who everybody called Doc. Karen really wanted us to be there so we could meet people, share our experiences, and get more support for Alfred's work in Ghana. I was glad to be there, and Alfred was too. I knew he was pushing himself mentally and physically to take in everything he could on his trip, so I could sense it was wearing him down.

When Alfred went outside to catch his breath, I followed him. We hadn't had a lot of time together to just sit and talk, so it was nice to finally be alone. The weather had cooled off, and a breeze had picked up. As we chatted, I could see his eyes beginning to close, and he was struggling not to nod off. He apologized for being tired. We sat side by side in silence just enjoying this time together. I thought "I can't believe I am sitting next to my angel – the person who changed everything for me. It was a beautiful but surreal moment. I also realized he was exhausted, so I found Karen and suggested that we let him go back to his hotel and get some sleep.

The next morning, Karen and Alfred dropped me off at the airport at 5 o'clock, for my flight home. They were heading to Karen's farmhouse about two hours away in the Kansas countryside. While I was pretty sad to be leaving my newfound friends, I missed my family, and I knew my boys needed me.

"Make sure he eats," I told Karen, nodding toward Alfred. "He's too thin." I hugged them both and said my goodbyes, trying unsuccessfully to hold back my tears. The uncertainty of not knowing when, or if, I would ever see Alfred again was tearing at my heartstrings.

But eventually a second opportunity to see Alfred in Kansas City arose in 2018. Alfred was making the trip with Prof. Ahmed Nuhu Zakariah and Dr. Maxwell Osei-Ampofo, to learn American emergency procedures, so they could improve those services in Ghana.

When I arrived this time, the Uber driver at the airport asked me "What brings you to Kansas City?"

"How long do we have?" I laughed. "Probably 45 minutes or so," he answered.

When the Uber driver told me how long the trip would take, I launched into my 45-minute version of the story about my mother, her mental illness, Ghana, Alfred, and finding forgiveness through God. While life has not been easy, I have learned to love this journey I'm on and where it has taken me. Alfred knew that I had started working on a book, but we hadn't had much time to talk. This is his story as much as mine, so I really want his voice helping me share it with the world.

"Wow!" the driver said as we neared our destination. "You are the most interesting person I have ever had in my car. I can't wait to read your book one day!"

"Thank you," I said, sincerely.

I am an infant as far as matters of my religious faith are concerned. My lifelong odyssey with my troubled mother, along with my new-found friendship with Alfred, has led me to conclude that there really *is* a God. I am just beginning to comprehend that for me to be success-ful as a mother, a wife and in life in general, it is extremely important to for me to humble myself before Him when I ask for His aid and guidance.

I've learned that by praying to God, He can open doors that might otherwise remain closed to us. But that is not to say that if we simply pray to Him that God will hand us the answers to all our problems. Instead, God challenges us to so that we can learn and grow from each of our experiences.

God didn't fix everything that was wrong with my mother and our broken relationship. Instead, He chose to guide me along a path-way of enlightenment so I could better understand each situation. God doesn't always make things easy. I didn't understand this before, but now I know that God wants us to learn by meeting our challenges head on but with the benefit of His grace. This is how we grow as human beings.

Every day I'm learning more and more about how important it is to fulfill our obligations to God. When He bestows His blessings upon us, we must meet his gestures in kind. God has faith in us, and we must keep our promise of faith to Him.

Looking back on my life, I recognize God's hand in so many of the things that had happened to me and my family over the years. Shortly after returning home to California from Kansas City when I first meet Alfred I prayed to God and told Him that if His plan for my life was complete, I could be content with everything He had already bestowed upon me.

But something way down deep inside told me that God wasn't done with me yet. Throughout this entire odyssey it's uncanny how many times something wonderful had happened from out of the blue right after experiencing the darkest of episodes. So many, in fact, that I've lost count. I just thank the Lord for making them all possible.

So, that night as I drifted off to sleep, I put my faith in His hands, and wouldn't you know it, the next morning I received a Facebook message from Andrea Rangecroft, an award-winning audio producer based in London. She wanted me to do an interview with the BBC. Another chance to spread the message about Alfred and a clear example of God's grace touching my everyday life.

Everyone always asks me how this story will end. In some strange way, I hope it never really comes to a close. I firmly believe that I will see Mom again in the next life, and she will be free from all the burdens that haunted her in this life.

As for myself, I hope to live in a way that will make both my Mom and Dad proud of who I have become. I want to be a good mother to my boys and a good wife to my husband. I want to show my sons that I am a strong person who possesses a genuine compassion for others just like Alfred does for those around him. I hope that my story will inspire others who are struggling with similar challenges in their lives, so that they can find inner peace.

I hope to continue shining a light on the important work that Alfred is doing in Ghana. One of the next steps in my journey will be to travel to Ghana to see Alfred, who I consider a brother, and meet his amazing family. I truly feel C, and their girls are part of my own family now. I hope to meet the other people in Africa who have done so much to influence my life and visit the place where Mom spent her last year.

I know God has a plan for each of us, and I am just starting to glimpse of what His plan is for me. I hope that I will have the grace and strength to face whatever challenges He has waiting for me.

Acknowledgements

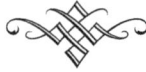

Ray Hemman, Liz Peters, Lynn Ischay, Richard Alan Hannon, Lou Loescher-Junge, Julie Mah and Brian Baresch. Without the help and guidance of this group of people this book may not have come about.

The Storytellers

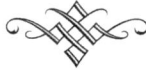

Katie Stakolich lives in Northern California where she and her husband, Rob, are raising their two sons, Ryder and Mason. A lifelong Californian, she has worked at the same grocery store for the past 25 years. She also dabbles in antique furniture restoration.

Katie says even though it has been a few years since her mother died, each time she reflects on of her mom's struggle with mental illness feels like watching someone else's life story unfold on an episode of Dateline.

Dr. Alfred Aidoo is a specialist anesthesiologist at Komfo Anokye Teaching Hospital (KATH) in Kumasi, Ghana, where he has practiced medicine since 2007.

In 2018, Alfred traveled to the U.S. on a fellowship sponsored by the American Association of Respiratory Care. In January 2022, he was selected to serve on Ghana's Pharmacy Council Board, which is tasked with ensuring drug availability, safety and regulation of the practice of pharmacy.

Alfred is an ordained reverend, and he and his wife have two daughters.

www.ingramcontent.com/pod-product-compliance
Lightning Source LLC
Chambersburg PA
CBHW030942090426
42737CB00007B/509